THE P★RN ANTIDOTE

ATTACHMENT:
GOD'S SECRET WEAPON
FOR **CRUSHING PORN'S GRIP**,
AND CREATING THE LIFE AND
MARRIAGE YOU DREAM OF.

CARL STEWART, MA

www.theporntantidote.com

ISBN-13:978-1530068142
ISBN-10:1530068142

www.thepornantidote.com
www.tpantidote.com

TABLE OF CONTENTS

ACKNOWLEDGMENTS

I am so thankful to my Lord and Savior Jesus Christ for the opportunity to serve Him as I get to see men be set free from pornography and marriages restored. Thank you to my amazing wife Julie- your support and encouragement as I chase my dreams is incredible...you are a blessing. Thanks to all of my friends and colleagues for supporting and encouraging me as well- I am blessed to have all of you in my life. Finally, thank you to all of the men, marriages, and families that I have been privileged to work with. What I have learned from you I am passing on to others.

INTRODUCTION

Pornography is shredding men, marriages, and families. This virus is spreading faster than you can imagine and it is affecting you whether you realize it or not.

Please hear me out - this not an overstatement or embellishment.

The facts speak for themselves:

According to the Barna Group (Survey, 2014):

* ✱ *79% of 18-30 yr old men.

* ✱ *67% of 31-49 yr old men.

* ✱ *49% of 50-68 yr old men.

* ✱ *55% of all married men

LOOK AT PORN ONCE A MONTH!

63% of adult men viewed pornography in the past three months at least once **while at work.**

THE P✱RN ANTIDOTE

"Sex" is the #1 searched topic on the internet.

Playboy stopped publishing pictures of naked women.

Think about that!!!

The CEO of Playboy told the New York Times:

> _"You're now one click away from every sex act imaginable for free. And so it's just passé at this juncture."_

If someone in your home isn't struggling with porn, then someone involved with your family certainly is. Your kids' friends (who all have iPhones with no internet filters), a neighbor, coach, or pastor - you are already rubbing elbows with guys who are knee-deep in porn.

This is the culture we live in, and we need a plan of attack. The virus is spreading.

This book dissects pornography and shows you how to truly defeat it. After reading it, you will have a clear understanding of:

* _How porn really works;_

* _How it hijacks your brain;_

* _The real reason you keep going back after you have sworn on your mother's grave to never look again (Hint: It's not just lust)._

I emailed a draft of THE P*RN ANTIDOTE to a pastor who came to see me.

He replied:

"Thank you for sharing this with me. Part of me said you wrote this after I left your office because it describes me so well, but I know that it was written long before we met. I must admit, yesterday I told myself I wasn't coming back be cause I felt better and finally telling someone my secret and I felt I could 'take it from here' and get better. But after reading those 10 pages those thoughts vanished."

Like a grenade going off in the home, pornography affects those around you. The information you are about to read will finally make sense of why your wife is so wounded, and it will show you how to repair your marriage.

If you don't know how this stuff really works, you may as well be walking through a minefield while blindfolded.

A wife whose husband had been deeply involved in sexual addiction read the first few chapters of THE P*RN ANTIDOTE and said,

"...I can see that glimmer of hope you are offering that so many need in a time of desperation and hopelessness....thank you for sharing your giftedness in saving our marriage..."

Another wife wrote:

"For many women who are newer in this mess (or men who have never understood why they turn there!) this will be EYE OPENING....there are root issues and that is what you do here - you explain the path to the behavior!"

THE P*RN ANTIDOTE deals with the root issues in a way that draws you more deeply into a relationship with Christ and others. The guys I work with in my private practice keep coming back to tell me that "LOOKING AT PORN DOESN'T MAKE SENSE ANYMORE!!!"

That is freedom. That is victory.

90% of my private practice as a counselor involves working with guys who are dealing with pornography/sexual addiction, and their marriages. I get the privilege of watching these men being set free, and seeing their marriages restored.

In fact, they are more than merely restored - the marriages end up better than both spouses could have imagined. That is a far cry from just "limping along" forever. It is amazing to watch the Lord exchange beauty for ashes and joy for mourning.

THE P*RN ANTIDOTE allows me to share all of the principles and truths that have been transforming people's lives in front of me for years now. I want you to be able to say what I hear guys tell me every week: "Porn doesn't make sense anymore," "It isn't a battle like it used to be," "I feel like a huge weight has been lifted - I don't have to hide anymore!"

Your wife will be relieved to finally understand why porn is so powerful for you when it doesn't make sense to her at all.

You will find hope for your marriage where you have previously felt terror and despair. You will see that your marriage can not only survive, but thrive! Repeatedly couples tell me that they are incredibly thankful for the marriage they have now - how it is better than anything they would have dreamed of before. They tell me it was a rough road to walk, but that it was worth it!

That is what I want for you. This is what the Lord has in store. What the enemy intends for destruction, the Lord intends for good. And the Lord likes to show off.

If you apply only 10% of what you read in THE P*RN ANTIDOTE you will see significant changes in your struggle with lust and porn, in your marriage, and in your relationship with the Lord. You will make the transition from resisting porn, to protecting a life that you love.

Don't put this off. Don't wait until you have "more time" to read this material and put it into action.

There is probably a voice in the back of your head screaming at you to run away from this book right now. The longer you run the harder it becomes to start. It is time to at least take a peek at something that will help you find freedom and peace.

If you have repeatedly fallen in the face of temptation and are telling yourself (again), "This time I mean it!! I can do this on my own!" please, save yourself the guilt and shame of falling again and wishing you had already done something.

Heed the words of these guys who did just that after years of trying and failing to quit on their own:

> "Carl and Christ helped save our marriage. Working with Carl gave my wife and I the tools to better love each other. When we first met Carl my wife was drowning in pain. We are now closer than we've ever

been and this closeness is running over to improve our whole family. Carl has been a great guide to reveal what Christ wants for us. Thanks Carl."

"(Carl) taught me that Satan uses my guilt to show me my past sins and tries to convince me that is who I am; Christ however sees a blank slate. Carl taught me that Christ actually wants to hang out with me; He is not just part of a Grumpy God that sits high in heaven and is too busy to deal with my small stuff. Christ wants to not only be my savior and king, but he also wants to walk through life with me."

"There is no magic cure, only God can completely heal you; however, this book has given a new hope. This book really helped me understand the addiction like I have never understood before."

Please turn the page now. Don't spend another day spinning your wheels and doing the same old dance that leaves you stuck in shame and despair.

Read the first two chapters- if what they say isn't transforming then put it down. Take this opportunity to change your trajectory.

See you in the next chapter.

CHAPTER 1:

Porn Is An Epidemic

Go to www.thepornantidote.com
for additional resources

Pornography is an epidemic. You heard that right - it's not just a 'growing problem.' Not a 'passing phase.' We live in a sexually saturated culture that is the perfect incubator for this virus. If you don't think it is a problem or affecting your life right now, then your head is in the sand and you need to wake up.

Unfortunately, porn is an epidemic in the church as well. How many Christian leaders have you seen go down in the media? How many pastors do you know of that lost their jobs, or at least their influence, due to "sexual indiscretions"? How many marriages and families do you know of that have been rocked by porn? Lost jobs, lost marriages, kids that insist on finding porn. This is the stuff I work with in private practice as a counselor in "THE MOST PORN LOVING RELIGIOUS CITY IN THE COUNTRY" (as per a porn distributor that compared visits to their website per capita from cities that rate themselves as religious or highly religious in the U.S. census data, on Buzzfeed.com). Yep, Huntsville, AL is #1.

I see the carnage - and the healing - every day. That is why I am writing this book - to give you what I share with guys and couples that leads to freedom. The strategies and principles I am about to share with you are what I use with folks that pay me a lot of their own money. My clients pay the full cost of counseling out of their own pockets, so if what I teach didn't work, they wouldn't keep coming back.

First, you have to look at the carnage. You have to see how big and bad the problem really is before you can understand why it's so important to tackle the issue.

Consider these statistics:

* ✱ 43% of internet users view pornography
* ✱ 25% of all searches are for pornography
* ✱ Sex is the #1 searched topic on the internet
* ✱ 35% of all downloads are pornographic
* ✱ 53% of Promise Keepers viewed porn in the past week
* ✱ 37% of pastors admit that they struggle with pornography
* ✱ Porn revenue is greater than all professional football, baseball, and basketball franchises

combined. (There is a ton of free porn available-so it is huge that people are willing to spend that much money on it!)

* 56% of all divorce cases involve one person with an obsessive interest in pornographic websites

* 69% of the pay-per-view market is pornographic

* 90% of 8-16 year olds have viewed pornography - most while doing homework

* 8 is the average age of first exposure to pornography. (The brain isn't ready to process sexual experiences until puberty.)

Think about those stats for a minute. This is happening in your neighborhood, your office, and your church. According to the statistics, it has been in your house.

The porn industry has changed since I was kid. It used to be that somebody had to steal a magazine from their dad. You had to actively look for porn.

Today, the porn industry seeks you out. It is aggressive and effective. Unsolicited email and pop-ups were just the start. This industry now targets website names that sound like the names of popular children's characters in order to lure kids in as young as possible. Consider 'www.barny.com' vs 'www.barney.com.' One is an annoying purple dinosaur that is crack cocaine for kids. The other is crack cocaine for adults. The former wears off a lot quicker.

Today's porn is powered by the 3 A's:

Affordable: Most porn is available for free. YouTube can't monitor the thousands of uploads per day. Revenues for the porn industry are declining due to so much free pornography offered on the internet.

Accessible: Every 5th grader has an iPhone. Few have a filter or are checked by their parents. Fifty percent of the time porn is viewed on a mobile device. Our school system issues computers to each student. Bless their hearts - they try to put filters on the computers, but any kid that wants to can beat the system. The kids I work with tell me all the time how they use school computers to access pornography. Then there is the computer at your desk...work cubicles still offer just enough privacy.

Anonymous: You don't have to go to the "bad part of town" to get this stuff. No more going to the room at the back of the video rental store. You don't even have to go to the corner gas station. Anyone, anywhere, anytime has a voluminous library of erotica readily available without the fear of being seen or recognized. What's to stop you?

This is typically what I hear when I challenge the widespread use of porn: "It isn't harming anyone," "All guys do it, so what's the big deal?" and "I look every now and then, who doesn't? That doesn't mean I have a problem." "It's natural, we are made to be sexual, so it can't be a problem." My first job out of graduate school was working in a residential drug rehab for teens. The minimizing, deflecting, and flat out denial sound all too familiar.

If you have looked at porn (or been to a massage parlor for a happy ending, gone to a strip club, been with a prostitute or girl from a "dating service", etc.), and felt regret, shame, or the need to hide the behavior, then you have a problem. If you go back to these behaviors, and these behaviors escalate over time, then you have a problem.

See if these types of guys sound familiar.

The Binger: You may have days, weeks, or months (sometimes a year or two) without looking or acting out. But then the urge hits you and you dive in head first, spending hours and days consuming as much porn as you can. Late at night after your wife goes to bed, or when she is out of town are prime times for you. Just knowing that you will have access and no accountability gets the juices flowing. Resistance seems futile. The fact that there are times when you don't look or act out provides a sense of control. "See, I can stop whenever I want," you might think. If you keep having to 'stop,' that means you haven't stopped...you've just paused.

The Compulsive: This person knows they cannot stop and they have no desire to try. If they attempt to stop, they know they won't in the end, so why bother? He is constantly thinking about sex and where to get his next fix. Thoughts of sex and erotica dominate his thinking throughout the day and this interferes with every aspect of his life. His reasoning goes something like this: "Why stop if it feels good and you know you will come back anyway?"

The Persistent Drip: This guy may binge occasionally, but his defining characteristic is that he looks on some sort of regular basis. Every few days, a few times a month, even a few times a year. It is not planned that way. For example, he looks a bit a work, maybe at night after his wife has gone to bed or when she leaves town. It isn't all the time. There is an ebb and flow to it. He will realize that he is spending too much time looking at pornography and abstain for a while. He is not surprised when he looks again. He may feel a sense of pride or control since it doesn't "seem" to control him. Again, he keeps stopping and convincing himself he has everything under control.

A lot of these guys feel guilty and mad at themselves after giving in. They swear they will never do it again. They put the filter back on, start exercising or embarking on some other self-improvement campaign, and for heaven's sake-don't tell anyone. "This time will be different," they tell themselves. Somewhere inside they know it will not work, and the pattern repeats itself.

Sporadic: This guy seems a bit more random. He has some traits seen in the other types. He will binge at times, be persistent at times, compulsive at others. Since there is no pattern, he wrongly believes that he doesn't really have a problem.

If you are reading this and wondering if you or someone you know has a problem, use the checklist below created by Robert Weiss M.S.W., C.A.S.

CYBERSEX ADDICTION CHECKLIST

If you answer yes to 3 or more questions, this may be an area of concern and should be openly discussed with a friend or family member.

If you answer yes to more than 6 questions, consider

(a) Counseling with a professional trained in addictive disorders

(b) Checking out a 12-Step support group for sexual addicts.

THE P✱RN ANTIDOTE

1. Are you spending increasing amounts of online time on sexual or romantic intrigue or involvement?

2. Have you been involved in romantic or sexual affairs?

3. Do you prefer online sex to having "real" sex with your spouse or primary partner?

4. Have you tried unsuccessfully to cut back on the time you spend online in sexual and romantic activities?

5. Has the time you spend on online sex or romance interfered with your job or other important commitments?

6. Have you collected a large quantity of Internet pornography?

7. Have you engaged in fantasy online acts or experiences which would be illegal if carried out (e.g. rape or sex with children or adolescents)?

8. Has your online sexual or romantic involvement resulted in spending significantly less time with your spouse/partner, dating life, or friends?

9. Have you lied about how much time you spent online or the type of sexual romantic activities you experience online?

10. Have you had sexual experiences online that you wish to keep secret from a partner or spouse?

11. Have your family or friends increasingly complained or been concerned about the amount of time you have spent online?

13

12. Do you frequently become angry or irritable when asked to get off the internet or computer?

13. Has the computer become the primary focus of your sexual or romantic life?

Source: *Robert Weiss, M.S.W.,C.A.S.*

Truthfully, if you answered yes to any of these statements you have an issue with porn. The question is how big will the problem get, and how bad will the consequences will be. Ignoring an infection is not a good plan. Do something before it grows.

In the next chapter I will clearly describe the mechanics of porn: How and why it is so effective. Later I will discuss the impact on wives and marriages. This is messy, but there is hope. Conventional wisdom says that the man with a problem should work on his recovery (for 6 months or a year), and then address the marriage. In my experience, this approach is marital suicide. I will tell you why, and what you need to do instead.

I will address the need for filters and accountability. These are necessary, but not sufficient. Like using a garden hose on a house fire, you will need to take a more aggressive approach to end the problem once and for all. I'll tell you what really works to put out the fire and heal the damage. It is amazingly effective. This is why I have guys in my office repeatedly telling me, "Porn just doesn't make sense to me anymore...it isn't a fight." That is victory.

What I am sharing with you is based on years of research and training. Research has clearly revealed that not all approaches are created equal. Neuroscience has taught us how porn affects the brain, why his brain is affected more than hers, and how to most effectively attack the house fire in a way that really works.

I began college as an engineering student. I could have been an engineer like my dad and everyone else in this city, but that was not my calling. However, this training taught me to analyze how things work, and not simply to accept someone's personal theory or flighty ideas. A client once called me a "social engineer." The fact that engineers keep coming to me to address emotions, relationships, and behavior says a lot.

Get ready - next I'll break down the mechanics of porn. Knowing how it works changes everything.

CHAPTER 2:

The Three Brains

Go to www.thepornantidote.com
for additional resources

Porn seduces with a promise: "This is what you want,"
"This will make you feel good," "This will make you feel
like a man." It promises everything you think you want in that
moment without showing what it will cost you later. By the
end of this chapter you will understand why we fall for the
trap so easily.

The same scenario played out in the Garden of Eden. Adam
and Eve didn't want for anything and sin had not yet
corrupted the world. There was no sadness, fear, or
heartache. So what happened?

They were seduced by the offer of "More." The offer of being
like God seemed too good to pass up. 'What could go

wrong?' they thought. After one bite the cost of "More" hit them like a ton of bricks. We have been experiencing the consequences and trying to hide our nakedness ever since then.

Porn is the apple offered to every guy. One bite...it won't hurt anybody, right?

Pornography hijacks the male brain. (More on why it doesn't do this to the female brain in a bit.) The male brain literally lights up when it sees something sexual. The MRI readout of a guy's brain when he is looking at pornography looks like a volcano exploding. The female brain, meanwhile...nothing. You can hear crickets.

The "3 Brains" theory explains why pornography acts like a drug. No, you do not have three different brains. These three parts of your brain interact with each other in a powerful way. Clients frequently tell me that understanding this dynamic has been pivotal in their recovery.

THINKING BRAIN:

The thinking brain is the prefrontal cortex. It is located at the front and top of your brain. If you have ever felt stupid and slammed the palm of your hand on your forehead, you hit the prefrontal cortex.

The thinking brain processes cause and effect, goals, morals, and values. It helps us apply what we have learned from our past experiences. When you are calm, this part of the brain works pretty well. When you feel a sense of connection with someone you love and care about, it is supercharged (you will hear a lot about this later).

When you we feel upset, afraid, or overwhelmed the thinking brain checks out. In that moment, you are not considering goals, morals, values, cause and effect, or your past experience – in other words, all of the checks and balances that God put in place. When the thinking brain checks out we are capable of doing just about anything.

The thinking brain isn't fully developed until age 25, and it is the last part of the brain to fully develop. This explains why car insurance is so expensive before the age of 25.

FEELING BRAIN:

The feeling brain involves several parts of the brain (known as the "limbic system") including the amygdala, and is located in the middle of the brain. The feeling brain is always evaluating whether you are safe and working to detect threats. It processes physical threats and emotional or relational threats in the same way.

In other words, if you hold a gun to my head or if my wife says she is leaving me I will feel the same way. Both possibilities are terrifying.

The feeling brain processes emotions, relationships, and, you guessed it, sex. In fact, the part of the feeling brain responsible for processing sex is two times larger in men than in women. This isn't an excuse for looking or lusting, but it gives some needed context.

In women, the part of the brain responsible for processing relationships is twice as large as the male counterpart. Guess what women spend more time thinking about?

We pride ourselves on our logical and rational culture. We are proud of our thinking brains. The problem is that our brain processes information through the feeling brain before the thinking brain gets to weigh in. Why? The feeling brain is here to make sure we are safe before we engage in analysis and reflection.

If the feeling brain determines there is a significant physical/emotional/relational threat, it takes the thinking brain out of the equation.

If a screaming man is charging towards me while slashing the air with large knives, I don't need to spend time reflecting and considering all of the possibilities. I don't need to think deeply about what is happening: "Is he a Japanese steakhouse chef?" "Is he being attacked by bees?" The reflective functions of the thinking brain are not what I need to be using in that moment.

There are a lot of connectors going from the feeling brain to the thinking brain. However, there are not many connectors going from the thinking brain back to the feeling brain. This is why it is hard to think your way out of being upset or overwhelmed. How many times have you said or done something when you were upset and regretted it later? Usually we say, "What was I thinking!?!" Truthfully? You weren't thinking at all.

Consider the experience of going to a haunted house. You know that people are going to try to scare you. You know that you will be just fine at the end. You can see people leaving who are laughing and have not been hurt at all.

You hear people screaming inside the haunted house even though they know they will not be harmed. The time lapse between the feeling brain and thinking brain allows you to experience the rush of fear before the thinking brain kicks in to remind you that it is all make-believe.

When the feeling brain perceives there to be a threat it automatically goes into some version of fight, flight, or freeze. If someone yells "GUN!" in a theater, you will be moving before you have time to think about it, or you will freeze to avoid drawing attention.

BODY BRAIN:

This is the brain stem, located on your neck at the base of your skull. This part of the brain is responsible for all of your bodily functions: Heart rate, breathing, blood pressure, etc. It is fully functioning at birth which allows us to live without having to think about blinking or breathing, which would be exhausting.

The brain stem mobilizes the body based on the perceived needs at the time. When everything is calm, it takes its orders from the thinking brain. When a threat is perceived, the feeling brain moves into the driver's seat. In that case the body brain gears up the system for fight, flight, or freeze.

There are a lot of connectors going from the feeling brain to the body brain. Similarly, there are lot of connectors going from the body brain to the feeling brain. This is where your "gut feeling" comes from.

When the feeling brain is processing something that has not been reflected on or analyzed by the thinking brain, yet the intensity of the feeling brain is transmitted through the electrical circuitry of the body brain, you experience a sensation known as a "gut feeling," because we typically feel this in our gut.

The two large vagal nerves descending from the body brain into your torso connect to all of your vital organs. These are the culprits for "getting butterflies" before a game or feeling nauseous when your team loses the big game.

Just because you have a gut feeling does not mean it is correct. It does mean the feeling or perception is worth investigating by using your thinking brain. Malcolm Gladwell describes this well in his book *Blink*. Gavin De Becker does an amazing job of fleshing this point out in his book *Protecting the Gift* (every parent should read it).

So what does all of this have to do with pornography? Everything! Let's look at how pornography hijacks a guy's 3 Brains.

When guy looks at pornography, the feeling brain (where we process sexual stimuli) lights up. Dopamine (the "gotta have it" drug produced by the brain) and testosterone levels surge when guys see something sexually stimulating. Dopamine encourages us to stay focused on sex, which causes the brain to release more testosterone, which in turn cues the brain to look for more sexual stimuli and the release of more dopamine. This is a powerful feedback loop - a snowball rolling downhill that gets out of control fast.

Just to make it even more fun, this feedback loop causes serotonin levels to drop. In guys this is experienced as tension or anxiety while simultaneously making you obsess on what is sexually stimulating you. This sexualized tension is screaming for a release.

Remember, when the feeling brain lights up, the thinking brain checks out. The part of the brain focused on goals, morals, values, processing cause and effect, and learning from past experience (i.e. when looking at porn has caused problems in the past), is not readily accessible. The part of the brain that would say "STOP! DON'T DO IT! THINK ABOUT YOUR WIFE AND YOUR JOB!" is being sidelined.

The dopamine release ensures that the tension feels really good and makes you crave more. Remember, the feeling brain and body brain are well connected. Since the sexualized feeling brain is giving the orders, the body is preparing for sex. Pulse and heart rate increase, hormone levels surge, you have an erection and are aware of the nerve endings in the penis that are screaming for stimulation.

This feedback loop rapidly escalates and consumes your whole mental and physical experience. In this moment, all of the rest of life fades away. You are not aware of the bills, your boss, your marriage, or your insecurities. All of life shrinks down to a very pleasurable and intensely sexualized experience that you are in "complete control" of.

This is an amazingly powerful and effective escape from reality. This is what makes sex and lust addictive. You become addicted to the dopamine and the emotional escape. With these images seared into long term memory for ready access, you can get a hit simply by recalling them any time.

The grand finale is when you act out on what your body has been ramping up for. This is sex with yourself (masturbation) or someone else. When you ejaculate your brain releases natural opiates like oxytocin that calm everything down. After super stimulating the feeling brain, oxytocin shuts down all feelings of tension for a while. Peace and calming...until the guilt and shame kick in. In that moment, all of life's problems go away. You are mentally and physically tension free. Again, until reality kicks back in.

Oxytocin is called the "cuddle hormone." It is responsible for causing us to feel attached to other people. At birth, the mother's body pours oxytocin into her system, creating a powerful bond between mother and child. Moms also get a good dose of oxytocin while breastfeeding.

Guys experience the greatest release of oxytocin after sex. We receive a lot more oxytocin than women after sex so it is understandably a lot higher on our agenda than it is on theirs. This means that whatever you "have sex with" you are bonded to. You can literally create an attachment to pornography. Be careful who or what you share oxytocin with.

As you can see, porn and lust are mood altering experiences. The fact that you can look at sexy pictures and make all of your problems go away for awhile is what makes porn addicting. The escape from reality by chemically overriding the brain is inherently addictive when left unchecked.

The more you engage in this mood altering cycle, the less effective it is. Less dopamine is released, so you have to find something more stimulating to get the same effect. Just like drinking alcohol consistently helps you develop a tolerance, requiring you to drink more to get the same effect, looking at pornography consistently means you have to find something more extreme to feel aroused. With drugs and alcohol, you have to put something in your body. With porn it is always one click away, or readily recalled in vivid detail from your memory bank.

Given that exposure to illicit images and videos is overwhelming for adult brains, imagine what it does to the adolescent brain. During adolescence the brain is two to four times more sensitive to the effects of dopamine. Everything is so extreme for kids during this period, and dopamine sensitivity is the culprit. What we think is kind of cool or interesting, they experience as totally amazingly over-the-top awesome. Therefore, they crave more of whatever made them feel that way. Dopamine junkies, the lot of them.

Remember, their thinking brains are still cooking until age 25. So adolescents are even more compromised when porn hits them. It's like they are shooting up with crack cocaine. Hearing the thinking brain in the midst of such overwhelming stimulation is like standing behind a 747 and trying to hear someone whisper. Good luck with that one.

Adolescents also don't feel the effects of excess as much as adults. They can keep binging and not experience the same "hangover" feelings experienced by adults. When it comes to their ability to handle pornography, the deck is stacked against them.

Kids that are exposed to pornography before adolescence are hit hard in a different way. (Remember, the average age of first exposure is eight years old). Developmentally speaking, this is a latent period (ages 8-11) where they aren't really interested in dating and their focus is primarily on playing and just being kids. Their brains are not ready to deal with sex yet. When kids encounter porn they are overwhelmed by the experience, their hormones spike and they feel sexually stimulated in a way they have not experienced before. Inherently they know this is something they are not supposed to be seeing so they hide, just like the child who hides in his room with the cookie he stole from the kitchen.

This hiding behavior means the child must deal with the confusion and stimulation alone. This dynamic makes the whole experience more stimulating, confusing, and shameful. The groundwork has been laid for a lifetime of hiding when things get overwhelming, confusing, painful. This is the story the men share in my office every day. This is the seedbed of sexual addiction.

I will talk more about the emotional triggers leading guys to escape into porn in the following chapters. Now that you have a framework for how the brain functions and how porn hijacks the brain, it is time to dive into the what drives guys to go down the porn spiral.

CHAPTER 3:

Emotions Managed By Porn

Go to www.thepornantidote.com
for additional resources

Now that you know how porn hijacks the brain, let's dive into those emotions that send you looking for somewhere to hide. Remember, we process information through the feeling brain first, which has a lot of connectors running to both the thinking brain and the body brain. When your emotions are triggered, your body responds accordingly (even if you have "numbed out" the basic experience of emotions). Your thinking brain does not have so many connectors to the feeling brain, so it is hard to cognitively override the feeling and body brains. It isn't impossible, but it is very inefficient. It leaves you stressed and dissatisfied if this is your go-to option over time.

26

As guys, we hear "emotions" and think, "That's fluff, girl stuff, weak, illogical and irrational, all emotions do is make things messy. If Bruce Willis didn't feel or express an emotion in *Die Hard* then I don't need to feel it either."

Having come from a math, science, and engineering background, I am here to tell you that there is a logic and rationale to emotions. You can learn to read emotions like a programming language, just like Neo in *The Matrix*. When the logic makes sense, you know how to respond. In fact, you can tap into the power that God put behind these emotions. (We'll get into that in the next chapter on attachment).

CONSIDER THESE EXAMPLES:

1. Robert has just been caught looking at porn by his wife. She found the history, looked over his shoulder, saw something on his phone...well, you get the idea. She is furious, crushed, and terrified. He is mortified, panicking, and in free fall. There is no quick fix for this situation.

2. Alan has been struggling with porn on and off for years and can not seem to completely cut it out of his life. He feels some degree of helplessness, hopelessness, or worthlessness because he can't "just stop". Alan is highly educated and logical. He may be former military. In fact, a lot guys that have been in or near combat have problems with pornography. They grow accustomed to being in a threatening environment and have a hard time shifting gears when they get home. They remain in a hypervigilant mode of being that has the body brain working overtime.

These two scenarios cover most of the calls I receive. The panic in these guys' voices is gut-wrenching. No matter how logical he thinks he is, emotions are driving him and he feels out of control. He wants help, and he wants it NOW!

It helps to think of emotions in terms of their intensity. The more intense an emotional experience is, the harder it is to manage. Imagine being in a pool of water with your feet tied to the bottom of the pool. If the water level (intensity) is at your armpits and some small waves come along it is no big deal. Nothing to stress about.

If these same waves come along when the water level is just beneath your nose, you are going to feel some stress. This is not necessarily overwhelming, but concerning. Your level of focus and vigilance go up, and your body is being prepared for fight, flight, or freeze. Remaining in this state for a prolonged period of time will cause you to oscillate between the feeling and thinking brain. Neither will be able to do their job well.

If the water level is at the bridge of your nose, you are already in an elevated state of fight, flight, or freeze. At this point, your thinking brain is not functioning well and all you can focus on is survival. Remember, it doesn't matter what caused the water level to get that high (a possible lay off at work, ongoing conflict with your wife, your team lost the big game...). Referring back to the examples above, Alan is probably in this state. The ongoing struggle and inability to stop leaves him in a state of despair.

If the water level is above your eyes, you can not tilt your head back to draw a breath. At this point you are in flat-out panic. If someone is threatening to kill you or your wife threatens to divorce you, this is what you will feel. This is where a lot of guys are when they call or come in to see me for the first time. This is Robert: Eyes wide open, feeling the pressure to fix things now or he will lose everything. It is rough.

Guys and couples I work with repeatedly tell me that referring to their "water level" is incredibly helpful. Simply acknowledging the intensity of your emotional or physical experience provides a clear idea of how overwhelmed you are. In turn, this tells others how available you are to hear or respond to them as well.

Couples tell me how simply telling each other where their water levels are helps them resolve a lot of fights, or even to avoid fighting altogether. Telling your spouse how stressed you feel in a way that makes sense helps them know if it is a good time to back off instead of push forward. "I'm stressed," a phrase these days synonymous with "I'm awake and breathing," is not as clear as "My water level is up to here!" (while pointing to their nose).

This is a clear "signal" (more on signaling in the next chapter) that I am getting overwhelmed and I need you to back off, or our conversation will not go well. It isn't personal, it isn't that I don't care about you or that what you are saying is unimportant. Because this signal is clear and communicates that I am not blowing you off, it is much more effective. Hearing that the someone is overwhelmed is a lot easier to handle than feeling blown off.

EXAMPLE 1

John and Laura (not a real couple; they represent a compilation of couples I have seen) have been married for years and are weary from "fighting all of the time." The following is a typical night in their home:

Laura is stressed from dealing with the kids, school, work, and keeping the household on track. John wanders in and asks Laura if she would pick up a prescription for him the next day.

Laura reels around with her eyes bulging and proceeds to unload in rapid-fire fashion everything that she is already doing. Her voice is loud and high pitched. "How can you ask me to do one more thing when I am already taking care of all of this!?!" (pointing to the kitchen table covered with papers and calendars.) Laura goes through the litany of tasks she accomplished today, what she wasn't able to do, and shrieks about how hopelessly behind she is for tomorrow. Her expression says, "I DARE you to ask me for something else."

John feels like he has been blindsided with a flamethrower. Confused, defensive, and now angry himself, John cannot understand how a simple question could set off such a firestorm.

As John gets defensive, Laura intensifies her response. They are off to the races. No-one wins. Both end up frustrated, hurt, and confused. Somebody is sleeping on the couch or in the guest room tonight.

John and Laura started using the "water level" idea as a way of communicating their stress levels to each other when things became tense. Here is how it played out with their new system in place:

Imagine the same basic scenario: Laura is busily working at the kitchen table, and John enters to ask for help with something. Laura reels around with her eyes bulging. In an obviously stressed voice Laura says, "My water level is up here" with her hand on her forehead like a salute, "And I can't think about adding anything else!"

John is stunned by the unexpected intensity. He is able to see and hear that Laura is overwhelmed. He doesn't feel attacked so there is no need for defensiveness or debate. At this point, John typically feels bad for Laura and offers to help. No-one ends up sleeping on the couch or in the guest room.

EXAMPLE 2

A family that I have been working with came in today and reminded me of how helpful the "water level" idea has been. I started working with the father who had a serious porn addiction before working with the marriage which needed a lot of repair. Then we started working with some of their kids that were having problems (including porn use). The husband, wife, and kids all said how useful it was to think in terms of "Where their own water/stress level is," and signaling (with their hand showing the water level) to each other.

The parents signal the kids, the kids signal the parents, the parents signal each other, the kids even signal each other. It's clear. It's simple. It's effective. No wonder guys like it.

Referring to water level opens the door for figuring out how stressed someone else is. Simply asking, "Is your level up here?" (with your hand somewhere around the nose), provides an effective escape route from unnecessary fighting and arguing. If we know someone is stressed and overwhelmed, we tend to give them time and space to settle down. It's like separating two guys starting a scuffle on Monday Night Football. You have to pull the guys apart and let them cool off.

Don't get me wrong, this family does not go around with their hands somewhere over their noses all the time in some kind of weird salute. Just know that referencing their water/stress level is a quick, efficient, and clear signal that helps prevent or stop a lot of unnecessary tension and fighting. It doesn't solve all of the problems, but it does prevent them from skyrocketing from bad to worse.

EXAMPLE 3

Another client I met with today - we'll call him 'Fred' - came in talking about his water level. Fred is highly analytical, and has been emotionally detached his whole life due to ongoing crisis and trauma at home while he was growing up. Mention 'emotion' to Fred and he looks at you like you are speaking Chinese. But 'water level' he understands. Fred was telling me how's he noticed his stress level at work and at home, showing where the water level was for each. Mr. Emotionally Detached quickly became fluent in describing his basic emotional experience. Fred's wife has been very thankful for this tool.

It's so easy even Dilbert could do it.

Stress is a universal language, which is why "signaling" by referencing water levels is so effective. However, there are significant differences between men and women that can drive these water levels up. If you don't know about these differences, then chances are you are inadvertently causing tension levels to rise.

NEWSFLASH: Men and women process emotions differently. Recall that the part of the emotional brain used to process emotional experience and relationships is twice as big in women as in men. Women typically have the edge when it comes to experiencing and expressing emotions. Discussing emotions is typically not as stressful for women as it is for men.

For men, being aware of emotions (besides "good" or "angry") is often pretty stressful. Guys are more likely to identify with terms like "intense," "stressed," "frustrated," or "overwhelmed" than softer terms such as "hurt," "sad," "inadequate," or "afraid." For a husband, having to discuss these emotions with a wife who is expressing her intense feelings with a lot of word power gets overwhelming in a hurry. Guys feel like they brought a knife to a gunfight.

The stress spikes and so does his water level. Guys use our "go to" emotional states: Shut down (called "stonewalling") or anger. This is called "flooding." When a guy is experiencing flooding, he has become emotionally and physically overwhelmed and his thinking brain has checked out. His heart rate shoots up, his blood pressure skyrockets, and adrenaline floods into the bloodstream. He gets angry and combative because he is just wanting the discussion to stop. Or he checks out (stonewalling). He mentally detaches, leaving his wife to literally talk to a stone wall.

Both responses have roughly the same physiological effects. A stonewalling response shows that what is happening is too stressful for him to deal with, not that it doesn't matter to him.

Once flooding has occurred, your chances of having a fruitful discussion are over. It will take at least 20-30 minutes for his body to regulate and be able to begin communicating about emotions or relational issues again. Wives have been dumbfounded to realize this. Guys have used this to perpetually avoid unpleasant conversations.

Interestingly, the tables are turned when it comes to a physical rather than emotional confrontation or threat. When you almost get hit by another car, she is more likely to be flooded. She is overwhelmed with what could have happened. She has a hard time shutting off the emotions and physically feels some level of fight, flight, or freeze. He feels fine - nothing actually happened, so what is the need for being upset? She feels wired for a while and can not stop thinking about the catastrophe they narrowly avoided.

Flooding is a trigger for a guy to seek the perfect escape in pornography. "Everything feels overwhelming...she doesn't understand me...she is unreasonable...I can't win...it's not fair...I know where to go to make all of this go away. I know what will drop the water level so that I can breathe again. I know what will make me feel good right now. I know what will make me feel wanted and powerful, even a way to get back at her," he thinks to himself.

The woman on the screen is always longing for you, affirming you. She never says no. She never gets upset. She never makes you feel like you can't win. What is happening on the screen, or even just a recollection of what you have seen, hijacks the brain and turns the tables.

Now the intensity is sexualized. Now you want more intensity. Now your thinking brain is more disconnected. Now you can act out and turn off all of the tension for a while. You hit the "Kill" switch. The more you do this the more you learn to avoid dealing with reality. The longer you avoid reality, the greater the consequences become. Hopelessness sets in as you perpetually escape into sexual fantasy and acting out. This leads to feelings of despair, and therefore more acting out. This nasty spiral only ends when you deal with reality.

Porn lures you deeper into the forest, promising that you can always deal with things "later."

Now let's look at the emotions driving this intensity. The very emotions porn is used to regulate, or flat-out bury.

A quick note on differences between men and women when it comes to managing emotional intensity. This may come as a shock, but the brains of men and women are quite different. No, this is not due to cultural influence, it is how God designed our brains to work.

First, the part of the feeling brain where we process relationships and emotions is two times larger in women than in men. In men, the part of the brain where we process sex is two times larger than in women.

Second, the part of the brain that connects the right and left hemispheres (the corpus callosum) is significantly larger in women than in men. The corpus callosum in a woman's brain is about as thick as a pencil. In men it is more like the width of the dot created by a laser pointer.

Why does this matter? The corpus callosum allows the left and right brain hemispheres to communicate. With fewer circuits connecting the right and left hemispheres of the brain, guys are inherently better at compartmentalization. I refer to this as "segmenting the hard drive."

As guys we can have an argument with our wives and later be surprised when they do not want to have sex. The "Emotional conflict" compartment is not connecting the dots with the "She's hot and I'd like to have sex" compartment. Segmenting the hard drive allows us to emotionally detach and focus on the task at hand. This skill is great at work, but not so awesome at home.

Women have exponentially more circuits connecting the right and left hemispheres of the brain. This explains why why everything is connected for her. For most women, compartmentalizing sounds as far fetched as Santa Claus. Because everything is connected, women are more likely to remember anything with emotional or relational significance.

Watch any mother leaving her kids with a babysitter - or better yet, grandparents - for a week, and your head will explode with amount of information and details (including how all of these details fit together). I am so glad my wife's brain keeps track of all of this information, our kids are probably alive because of it.

There is a down side. Women will also be able to keenly recall times where they have been hurt or let down. Their brains won't let them segment and ignore things like men. They think about it and think about it. This is where men accuse women of getting "historical."

According to Dr. Daniel Amen, at a resting state 90% of the female brain is activated. Think about that. 90% is her resting state. For the male brain, this figure is 30%. Her brain is processing, and processing, and processing. Therefore, women have a harder time shutting down and relaxing.

I have found that women, especially moms, typically have a harder time sitting still and being in the moment. My wife is thinking about what we need at the store, how one of her good friends is doing, how to help our kids with school, how to coordinate all of the schedules for our family, and the 2,364 emails that came in today. It wears me out just thinking about all that she is processing.

As a guy, I can turn on ESPN or a good action movie and the rest of the world goes away. Gaming does the same thing. Frankly, guys feel better knowing that women are thinking about all of the problems in the world. The unwise man who probably sleeps on the couch a lot says, "Sure I'll listen, but can you wait until the commercial to tell me about it?"

Guys do not understand why she can not "let it go." Women can not understand how we can simply not think about it. Mark Mungor has a great bit on this in his series, titled *Laugh Your Way to a Better Marriage*. This idea is also the premise of the book, *Men are Like Waffles, Women are Like Spaghetti*.

So how does this apply to sex or sexual addiction? Great question. When guys' brains spike to 90% with emotional conflict we are flooding. Women don't understand what the big deal is. They feel hurt, angry, and rejected when we bail out to keep our head from exploding.

Guys- this is not an excuse to avoid emotional conflict. It means she does not understand why the situation is so stressful for you. With flooding comes the pursuit of an escape hatch such as porn, which is effective and readily available.

Guys are typically in a sexually positive state, meaning we can be ready for sex at any moment. Women are typically not wired this way. They need help calming their brain down to somewhere near 90% to be interested, or aware of, sex.

This is more than, "You look hot." Your wife requires emotional engagement to help her brain wind down and feel good about being with you in the moment. She typically does not de-stress by having sex the way that a guy does.

Numerous guys have told me the same story. After getting married their sex life was pretty good. When kids came along it took a plunge. There was more stress, less time to connect, and more conflict. So he turns to pornography. Many times the guy feels angry, like he has been cut off and all that matters now is the kids. When the wife finds out that he has brought porn into the home with her kids she is enraged. Trust me, this is not good for your love life.

Life hack: Research shows that husbands who help around the house more have better sex lives. Start voluntarily doing some extra tasks around the house, without drawing attention to your efforts, and watch what happens.

CHAPTER 4:

The Logic Of Emotions

Go to www.thepornantidote.com
for additional resources

"Intensity" describes emotions from the thousand-foot
level. Now it's time to drop down for a closer look at
these feelings.

First, consider the logic of emotion. (No, this is not a
contradiction in terms.) Emotion is feedback. Rich,
necessary, and relevant feedback. Emotional feedback
shows what you really believe at a core level, as well as
what you need.

If I told you there is a huge rattlesnake on the other side of
the door in front of you, what would you feel? Because you
know this isn't real it is easy to dismiss. But if it were real,
you would probably feel some level of fear. The flash of

panic on the face of clients who are afraid of snakes is telling when I use this example.

The fear is not necessarily caused by the snake. It is caused by what you already believe about snakes, danger, threat, pain, death, etc. The beliefs manifest as emotions which cause you to take action. Emotion is the subjective experience that causes you to take action. In this case you might scream, freeze, barricade the door, or (in the case of my friends in Special Ops) grab a knife and have rattlesnake for lunch. I hear they taste like chicken.

Most of the folks I work with are Christians. In speaking with these guys I can tell there is a genuine love for the Lord and belief in His word. They have often taught others that God will provide all of our needs, and that we shouldn't worry about anything.

Then they get laid off. The panic about providing for their family and possibly losing the house reveals a competing belief that was there all along: "It's all on my shoulders to provide." Being emotionally triggered like this shows where the Lord is still working on us.

These same emotions reveal what we need. The deeper and more vulnerable emotions (stay with me guys, I know I mentioned "vulnerable" and "emotion" together) provide clearer indications of what we really need. Sadness shows we need comfort and to grieve. After losing the championship game on TV the losing team comforts their team mates who feel crushed.

Just as feeling hungry leads you to seek food, loneliness pushes us to seek connection with others. This is why lonely people go to a bar on Christmas Eve. Loss leads us to grieve. Fear leads us to seek security and protection.

As you will read later, your brain is hardwired to operate this way. Our brains are hardwired to pick up on these emotional signals from other people so that we know what they need, as well as how to respond. Emotional feedback is what we share with the Lord and with those we are close to. This makes us feel closer and calmer.

Connecting with the Lord and with others via these emotions actually regulates our emotions and physiology. Essentially, this turbocharges the thinking brain. You heard me - we do our best thinking and are most creative when we experience a sense of connection with Christ and others.

How does all of this tie in to pornography? As guys, we tend to avoid these types of emotional experiences. Pornography, lust, and acting out are processes that help mask and override emotions that seem overwhelming or out of control.

Experiencing the full depth of our emotions is not always the best idea in the moment. If you are in a combat situation, being debilitated by fear or sadness over the loss of the guy next to you isn't helpful. Likewise, watching your two-year-old ride his big wheel into the busy street into oncoming traffic (I actually did this) is not a time to be frozen with fear. In moments like these we need to be able to contain the emotional experience so that we can function, fight, and protect.

The "secondary emotions" of anger or numbness are what you feel when the entire bandwidth of an emotional experience is narrowed down to a more manageable sliver.

41

As guys we tend to gravitate towards anger or numbness because when we experience these emotions, we feel in control. Ask a guy how he is doing and you will probably hear "Fine", "Stressed", or "Frustrated." We will almost die before admitting that we don't have everything together.

Secondary emotions are there to help us function and get through a situation. However, staying in this mode leaves you feeling empty and dead after a while. Avoiding the messy emotions you don't want to experience while still feeling alive, requires an intense and overriding experience. This could be football, obsessive exercise, eating, or (you guessed it) porn.

Think about the high school kid stressed out by school, peers, and a rough home life. The CEO who is always wired and can't shut down. The soldier that has come home and is trying to keep everything he experienced from flooding him. The father who is trying to make his wife happy, pay for braces and travel ball, and keep up at work. You can see how easy it is for men in these situations to camp out in the secondary emotions of anger and numbness.

Secondary emotions are like football players getting Novocain shots in their knees in order to keep playing. It doesn't solve the problem, it just keeps you from being aware that there is a problem. The longer this continues the more damage it creates. A short term solution used for the long term creates long term damage.

It is time to go deeper. We started with emotional intensity, then secondary emotions. Now let's look at the emotional base of the pyramid: Primary emotions.

At the most basic level, the primary emotions behind anger and numbness are fear and pain.

I am afraid of my child being hit by a car, so I get angry which moves me to take action. Your team loses the game and you punch a hole in the wall because you are disappointed with the outcome and helpless to change it. Your wife discovered your porn again and you are terrified she will leave you. Numbing is a welcome escape.

Some experts make a big deal arguing over which emotions are the essential "core" emotions. They argue that some of what I describe here are beliefs rather than emotions. For academic theory and research that is great, but I am using emotional terms and descriptions that I have found are the easiest to connect with, especially as a guy.

Here is a good smattering of emotions that underlie most any experience: Joy, fear, sadness, shame, disappointment, helplessness, hopelessness, despair, inadequacy (a big one for guys), and worthlessness.

Anger can be a primary emotion, but most of the time is isn't. Anger as a primary emotion is about protesting against something unjust. Someone breaking into your car, punching your child, lying about you, etc. When Jesus tore apart the temple He was righteously angry. However, when we get angry, there is usually other stuff involved as well.

Honestly, most of the time my anger is not righteous indignation. Usually it is a result of my pride and insecurity. (Unless someone is going slow in the left lane, then anger is definitely a righteous response.)

So let's take a look at the emotions we stuff. The biggest hitter and the most toxic emotion that we have to deal with is shame.

Shame and guilt are different. When I feel guilty, I did something bad and I feel conviction and remorse about it. When I feel shame, I think that I am bad because of what I did. Shame is a death spiral that can easily ruin your life.

In my full-time private practice where I walk alongside guys fighting to get out of the porn rut, shame is the biggest block. We mask shame with anger. For example, your wife says you don't work hard enough, or puts you down. All you hear inside is your dad saying you are a slacker or will never amount to anything. So, you get angry at your wife, yelling at her for being unreasonable, irrational, and pointing out everything you have done to prove that you have not failed. To prove that you are not a failure.

Somewhere inside you believe that you can't keep up any of the successes you have earned. I work with guys that have started and sold multi-million dollar companies who are still trying to prove their worth. No matter how much success they have on the outside, they are weighed down with the millstone of shame hung around their neck along the way.

Pornography is a great anesthetic for shame and feelings of worthlessness. Porn makes these emotions go away when you are being crushed beneath their weight. Guess what one of the by-products of acting out is? You guessed it - shame. What a wicked and efficient cycle.

Sadness and loss are powerful emotional states that easily lead to escaping into the porn portal. Just this past week I met with a guy who went through a horrible divorce after his wife repeatedly cheated on him. In his current marriage, any time his wife gets upset or seems flirty with another guy it sends him over the top. The pain and anguish of what happened is so great it feels like she is cheating all over again. He is numbing out through porn before you can blink.

Right now you might be saying, "I'm not like that. I don't have problems with those feelings. I get frustrated, or a little down at times, but none of this soft mushy-gushy stuff applies to me." Please hear me out - just because you have not let yourself connect to these emotional states doesn't mean they aren't there. God created you to have these emotions for a reason (stay tuned for the next chapter).

I have been in my office with successful athletes, diehard engineers (rocket scientists are a dime a dozen around here), farmers, military Special Ops...you name it. The guys that you would think are least likely to feel or need these emotions. When we start digging into why they act out, what was happening emotionally leading up to their acting out, they are as surprised as anyone that they have these emotions and that these emotions have so much influence. I am honored that these guys are so transparent with me.

Mike sat in my office telling me how he is driven to succeed. Mike is the CEO of a rather successful company and has done very well for himself. "I can't turn it off," he says. Enough is never enough.

Mike feels burned out and self medicates with porn and alcohol. He played sports through college and was a stud on and off the field. Every guy would say that he has it made and should be completely happy and satisfied but no matter how great the achievement, Mike never feels like he has arrived. He never feels like he is truly successful.

After a little digging, he came to a stark realization. Mike's dad pushed him hard in everything he did. Nothing was ever good enough. Two homeruns in a game was not enough – he would say, 'You struck out on a bad pitch.' No matter how well Mike did, his father focused on the areas where he needed to improve. He internalized this and let it run his life. Mike wasn't succeeding because he wanted to. He was working so hard because his sense of worth and value depended on it.

Once this became clear, Mike did some work on these beliefs and feelings about his worth. He was able to work because he wanted to and was able to say no without feeling worthless or shameful. He didn't have to self-medicate. In the end, it was not a white-knuckle battle.

In my experience, there are three emotions that we cannot tolerate. We will do anything to get away from them. I call them the Devil's Triangle: HELPLESS, HOPELESS, and WORTHLESS. When I talk with guys and couples, these are typically the basis of their strongest emotional reactions.

Here's an example. Rob comes to see me because he has relapsed again and his wife is on the warpath. He is terrified that she will take the kids and leave him. He has tried everything he knows to do, really meaning it every time. Yet Rob ends up acting out again within six to eighteen months.

Rob feels helpless because he can't make himself stop for good. He feels hopeless. If he can't stop for good (which history now tells him that he won't) then everything meaningful to him will walk out the front door. Rob feels worthless because he realizes this is a self-inflicted wound. The shame is crushing.

At the same time, Rob's wife feels helpless since she can't keep Rob from going back to porn. She feels hopeless because it keeps happening. She can't imagine a future without this cycle. She feels worthless because "Rob obviously wants women that look like porn stars and do what porn stars do." Rob's wife feels like she can never measure up, that she is just not good enough.

When the Devil's Triangle of helpless, hopeless, or worthless (they typically come as a package deal) are evoked it is a "hair on fire" type of experience: Overwhelming, flooding, and panicking (fight, flight, or freeze).

It is hard enough when one spouse feels this way. When both spouses feel like this at the same time it can get ugly in a hurry. There is a chapter coming up on how to deal with the marriage when both of you have your hair on fire. Jump ahead if you need to.

Too often, the seeds for feeling hopeless, helpless, or worthless are planted early in life. Research shows that the best predictor for any type of addictive behavior is a history of abuse (physical, emotional, or sexual). Abuse is more than getting spanked as a child, or losing privileges over and over again. Abuse is demeaning and dehumanizing treatment that crosses the line from being painful or uncomfortable to destructive and damaging. It deeply affects the way you see yourself and others.

Craig's dad was an alcoholic who went into rages when he drank. Beatings were commonplace for Craig and his siblings (watching someone else receive abuse is traumatic as well). Anything Craig liked, his dad verbally attacked. He liked fishing – his dad said fishing was lame. If Craig got 5 A's and one B, his dad criticized him for the B.

Craig's mother felt guilty that she couldn't stop his father, and that she didn't protect Craig by leaving her husband. Feeling trapped herself she would confide in Craig about her own hurt and anger. She would frequently seek approval and affirmation from Craig about her looks, even asking if she looked sexy.

What both parents did is abusive in different ways. His dad's part is an obvious case of physical and emotional abuse. The message came through loud and clear: You will never amount to anything, you are never safe, and nothing you ever do will be good enough. Can you spot the well rooted seeds of helplessness, hopelessness, and worthlessness? If your dad repeatedly says these things about you while growing up, the message sinks in deep. It simply feels "normal" because it is what you experienced.

Craig learns to think the following: "If my dad thinks this about me, and he is supposed to love and protect me, how can I expect anyone else to love or protect me? Maybe I really am worthless." You would be surprised how many type A hard drivers have this type of experience at their core. No amount of "success" calms the emptiness and ache inside, so porn becomes a great way to self medicate and check out. Besides, the women on the screen are always smiling and affirming. That is intoxicating.

Craig's mom crossed some serious and destructive lines as well. A parent relying on a child for emotional and relational needs that should be met by a spouse is called emotional incest. Confiding in her son is something Craig, who was just a child, was not equipped to handle.

Adding a sexualized component creates a connection in Craig's brain between mom and inappropriate sexuality. Simultaneously, Craig felt important because he was able to help mom (lots of affirmation), and yet awkward about her "sexy" comments. Shame became connected with sex. What a fertile seedbed for sexual addiction.

Abuse is easy to spot, but often it is hard for folks to acknowledge that they experienced abuse. "Sure mom would get a little rough when she whipped us, don't all parents do that?" "Dad would blow off steam when he got home, but I know he loved me so it's no big deal." We don't want to think of those we love as being abusive, or that we were abused. It is confusing to sit with the reality that they loved you, and that they were abusive.

Neglect is the silent killer. While abuse is the best predictor of any type of addictive behavior, neglect is the best predictor of how persistent that behavior is. Neglect is when you don't get what you need. If you didn't get the big wheel you wanted when you were three, you were not neglected. Cutting off cable and removing sweets from the house is not neglect.

Parents refusing to set and keep healthy boundaries with kids is neglect. Craig experienced neglect from both parents: dad flat out refused to be involved in a healthy way in his life. No support, no mentoring, no guidance. Craig's mom didn't provide protection from obvious abuse, and she neglected his emotional needs to meet her own. Engaging her son in a sexual manner was abusive and incredibly confusing. I believe that neglect is so powerful because it is hard to pinpoint. It is like realizing you have an open wound and not knowing where it came from. Your experience is more confusing and out of control. The experience and beliefs of helplessness, hopelessness, and worthlessness come in below the radar.

Trauma is also highly associated with addictive behaviors. Trauma is more than just a bad day. It is an overwhelming emotional experience characterized by some combination of (you guessed it) helplessness, hopelessness, and worthlessness.

Being beaten by a parent, sexual abuse, death of a sibling or parent, a massive car wreck, watching buddies die in combat – all of these are typically traumatic. Since the brain is overwhelmed and not able to process the experience, it leaves a nasty footprint. In fact, the brain stores traumatic experiences differently than other memories. Since the original event was experienced as exceedingly overwhelming, we inherently never want to go through something like that ever again. Therefore, the brain supercharges the imprint on the emotional brain.

When this memory is triggered, you will re-experience the emotional intensity all over again. You may even have flashbacks (involuntary recall of the visual memory with the overwhelming emotions) of the original event as if it is happening again right now. Think of a Marine in Starbucks diving beneath a table when a car backfires. The emotional brain takes over and the thinking brain is offline. His emotional brain screams that someone is shooting at him.

Pornography is a powerful way to override trauma. It turns off the experience fear and anxiety in the emotional brain for a while. Yes, it causes other problems, but it provides a compelling "off switch." Craig would use porn to calm down after something triggered the thoughts and feelings of dad beating or demeaning him. Any sense that his wife was not totally pleased with him was enough to do this. Hijacking the brain with porn provides a powerful escape from emotions and heightened physiology (flooding) in the moment. The lingering effects create the very thing you are trying to escape - shame, helplessness, hopelessness, and worthlessness.

There are three other things to look for when someone is struggling with pornography or addictive behavior: ADHD, anxiety disorders, and bipolar disorder.

The three hallmark traits of ADHD are inattention, hyperactivity, and impulsivity. Impulsivity is acting before you think. We can all be impulsive at times.

However, the impulsivity from ADHD causes perpetual problems across different settings (work, school, home, etc). With ADHD, the filter needed to evaluate whether something is a good idea or not doesn't work so well. Therefore, people with ADHD have a harder time thinking through the temptation to look at porn because it is so very stimulating. ADHD compromises the thinking brain, which is already at risk for any guy exposed to porn.

Scott is an incredibly intelligent and creative engineer. He can be very logical but also very impulsive. Scott really loves the Lord and wants to stop looking at pornography. Unfortunately, he gets bored quickly and starts surfing the net on his phone.

While reading an article on a news site he notices an add on the side with a picture of a sexy woman (foxnews.com comes up in my office a lot for this reason). Scott clicks on the picture before considering if it is a good idea or what may happen next. Then he clicks on the next picture. He has gone down the rabbit hole before realizing what he is doing. Sometimes medication is a necessary tool to restrain the impulsivity. This gives guys like Scott a fighting chance to think through what they are doing.

Anxiety disorders are next on the list. We experience anxiety or stress as part of life. An anxiety disorder means that your anxiety remains heightened and is hard to bring it down. Anxiety is stress, fear, or worry that is out of proportion to the situation.

Some anxiety disorders simply keep you feeling perpetually stressed or anxious (which may present as agitation since this is a fight/flight/freeze emotion). PTSD falls in this category, as does generalized anxiety disorder, and O.C.D.

Anxiety is the response to a perceived threat, which is a function of the feeling brain. If the feeling of threat remains elevated, the body stays ramped up, and you wear down. We all look for relief from this kind of stress. Jogging or watching *Die Hard* with a pan of brownies has worked for me many times.

Because the feeling brain is already ramped up, porn can easily become a go-to escape. Remember, it overrides the fear response and calms that part of the brain down temporarily. It is truly an attempt to self-medicate.

Clark has O.C.D. He is a great worker because things have to be perfect. The stress gets to him every few days and he ends up looking at porn to escape. Once Clark comes back to his senses, he obsesses over how guilty he feels and how "bad" he is. This ramps up his emotions for the next episode of looking at porn (or drinking, or gaming, etc.). Treating an anxiety disorder with therapy and possibly medication is essential in these cases.

Bipolar (manic depressive) disorder is a tough one. We all have mood swings, but folks with bipolar disorder live on an emotional rollercoaster. It may be the old wooden roller coaster with some ups and downs that don't seem too far out of the norm (this is called Bipolar type II, kind of a "baby bipolar"). Type I bipolar disorder is the totally wicked awesome coaster that throws you around like a rag doll. Going from a euphoric state where you feel like you can do anything to the depths of depression and despair is brutal. After crashing into depression, pornography can become a welcome escape.

Bipolar is a biological issue and typically requires medication to keep it in check. These mood swings make you feel out of control, as well as hypersexualized at times.

Eric is an exciting guy to be around, the life and soul of the party. He makes everyone laugh and has boundless energy. Eric can also be angry and agitated, or simply drop out of sight for a while. When he feels up, he binges on porn and doesn't need much sleep. Porn helps him feel in control and regulate his emotions that have been taking him for a wild ride.

CHAPTER 5:

Attachment - The Secret Ingredient

Go to www.thepornantidote.com
for additional resources

Attachment is the secret ingredient that drives emotions, behavior, and physiology. It's is more than just a connection with someone. You can have that with a casual acquaintance.

Attachment is a bond, or the process of seeking a bond, with another person or group that goes much deeper. The bond between mother and child, husband and wife, best friends, two war buddies...these are all examples of a deep bond between two people. Every year athletes receiving the MVP award and those inducted into the Hall of Fame for their sport tearfully credit their moms (most often) and dads.

Award shows (the Oscars etc.) of full of stars thanking their spouses for their encouragement and sacrifice. You are constantly surrounded with examples of attachment. If you tune in to the music of attachment you will understand the dance everyone around you is doing.

God designed us to be attached to Him and to each other. Jesus said the greatest commandment is to love the Lord with all of your heart, and to love your neighbor as your self (Matt. 22:37-39). This is a deep level of loving. It is not convenient or easy. This type of love led Christ to suffer and die for us when there is no way we deserved it.

That is attachment. That is why we suffer for our children when all they do is eat, sleep, and poop. They have done nothing to deserve our love, yet we love them intensely and protect them ferociously.

We process attachment and relationships in the feeling brain. Remember, this is the part of the brain that is always evaluating safety or threat. When you have allowed yourself to become deeply attached to someone it is as if a ligament connects the two of you. This bond typically takes about two years to develop and is incredibly strong and resilient. Like steel cables, it can bend and contort without snapping whilst bearing massive amounts of weight.

This is where I usually get the questions about marriage. "If attachment is so strong, why is the divorce rate so high?" Please hold on to something sturdy, because I have some shocking news for you. You have been duped, I have been duped, we all have been duped. Not only is the divorce rate below 50%, IT NEVER HIT 50%!

The divorce rate spiked in the 1970s with the advent of "no-fault divorce." The divorce rate was projected to reach 50%, but a funny thing happened along the way. People realized divorce was not everything it was cracked up to be, so couples refocused their efforts on staying together and working things out.

The best estimate of the current divorce rate is 20-25% for first marriages, and 31% for all marriages (including first, second, third, etc.). Shanty Feldahn, a Harvard-trained researcher, thoroughly debunks the urban legend of the 50% divorce rate in her book, *The Good News About Marriage.*

This means that attachment is an incredibly strong and stable bond. These bonds can stand the test of extreme trials and survive more than we thought. Take heart if your marriage is on the rocks: there is more hope than you thought. This is great news if your marriage is in turmoil due to pornography or sexual addiction.

Being housed in the emotional brain, attachment generates intense emotions. A lot of physiological intensity, as well as the ensuing intense behaviors, are the result. Think about it. When you are attracted to someone and are developing a relationship with them, your thinking brain checks out. You have boundless energy and obsess about them. You want to see them, touch them, and hear their voice. How much sleep have you given up to be with someone you are in love with or are deeply attracted to?

I had a friend in college that would climb in his car and drive 12-15 hours just to get to see a girl he was infatuated with. He didn't need to sleep or eat much. All that mattered was getting to be with her and talking on the phone wasn't enough. It wore him out - and no, they did not get married.

These deep bonds have a life and death quality to them. If you hold a gun to my head, and my wife said that she wanted a divorce, I would feel the exact same thing. That is why attachment is so important to understand. It is both calming and reassuring. It also causes the deepest pain and fear imaginable. (Just ask a parent who sees their small child running towards the street, or parents of a 16-year-old who just received their driver's license and is out late for the first time). Nobody on this earth can make me feel more special and important than my wife, and no one can hurt me more deeply than my wife can.

Since attachment drives emotional and physical intensity, it is vital to understand how it works. After all, porn is a way of escaping and managing emotional and physical intensity. You are about to see precisely why attachment is the antidote to porn. Why attachment is the IOS - the Interpersonal Operating System.

From the last chapter, you know that there are three emotional states that quickly send us into panic: Helplessness, hopelessness, and worthlessness. When we feel this fear or panic we will either isolate or reach out for help from someone else. These are called attachment behaviors. One strategy is to become very intense and demanding so that others will either: A) Come close to help (like a drowning person flailing in the water, or B) Stay away because they are perceived as a threat (like a lion with a thorn in its paw).

Another strategy is to flee. Fleeing can be done with the intention of avoiding conflict altogether, minimizing conflict, or even lying to avoid the possibility of conflict (i.e. "if I tell her I looked at porn again she'll kill me, so I'll lie about it"). This is my natural tendency that the Lord has had to grow me out of. I can entertain you, make you laugh, and change the subject as needed to avoid tension and conflict. It is exhausting. A lot of guys I work with fall into this category. Their wives want to have difficult or stressful conversations and the guys feel terrified and overwhelmed. So they endure the interaction and use porn to self-soothe afterwards.

Finally, there is the freeze response. This occurs when you feel overwhelmed and it seems like your brain shuts down. You find it hard to think or possibly even move. In college I was walking around downtown Chicago with a friend. We passed by a Jeep with a German shepherd tied up in the back. Barking ferociously, the German shepherd lunged at me with teeth that seemed large enough for a dinosaur. The Jeep did not have a cover on it so there was nothing separating my face from the dog. The leash kept the dog from actually attacking me, but those teeth came within six inches of my face. My friend jumped away like a cat on a hot tin roof. I didn't flinch. He thought I was brave - tough as nails – but just the opposite was true. It startled and scared me so intensely that I could not jump. I could not think. This is a freeze response.

After freezing in the face of your wife, your boss, etc., you feel inadequate. (That is to say, you feel some form of worthlessness.) Porn becomes an attractive strategy to feel better about yourself (the girl in the picture looks at you like you're a stud), and overrides the emotions and physiology of shame and embarrassment.

Attachment is at the center of the bull's-eye. The purpose of emotion is to grab our attention and point us towards a safe connection with Christ and others. The physiological intensity is designed to get us moving to either find this safe connection, or get us away from unsafe connections with others. Attachment is the driver!

Let's crack the code of the Interpersonal Operating System a bit more. There are very specific attachment behaviors to look for in yourself and others. Your life will change dramatically as you learn to pick up on these behaviors. They provide a clear road map. Like Neo in *The Matrix*, you start seeing everything on a whole different level.

These attachment behaviors serve a number of purposes: Bids for connection, proximity seeking, attachment protest, and repair attempts. Fortunately this is a small list. I promise you, if you start seeing the "attachment significance" of these behaviors and responding to the meaning behind them (in yourself and others), your life will run smoother, you will have a lot more peace, and you will be happier than you ever thought possible.

At a marriage seminar a couple volunteered to be guinea pigs when we began discussing attachment behaviors. It came out that the husband loves going to Alabama football games. His wife could care less. The husband made a big deal out how much she needed to go with him. She pushed back, annoyed that he seemed to only focus on what he wanted to do. This changed when we looked at this through an "attachment lens." I asked why he wanted her to go, and what it was like if she did not accompany him to the game. The husband lit up with how much he loved going and how sharing this experience with his wife makes it even better.

She saw the sadness in his face, and heard it in his voice when he talked about going without her. Once she realized it was all about him wanting to share the experience with her because she was so special to him, her perspective did an about-face. She loved the idea of going to the game after that conversation. The ongoing fight about game day was officially over, and they both won.

The husband wanting his wife to go to the game is a "bid for connection." It is literally an attempt to connect relationally. It wasn't clear to her that he was really wanting to be with her, to connect with her, so she didn't see what the big deal was. When she did, everything changed.

Asking about your day, sitting down next to you, talking about what happened in your own day - there are thousands of ways that we try to connect with others that are not obvious. When they fall flat, we feel disappointed, hurt, or even angry.

It is easiest to see these behaviors in our kids. "Daddy look at me...," "Come play with me," "Read me a book," etc. When we pick up on the attempt to connect we are tuning in to the music, we know how to dance. Ironically, even if you can't take them up on the bid, affirming the desire to connect is almost as good. In such a situation, say something like, "I'd love to go out to eat - I love spending time with you. Unfortunately I promised our neighbor I would help him with his dryer tonight." Research shows that picking up on the intent to connect is vital, just like the wife picked up on her husband's intent to connect by going to the football game.

Simply turning your attention towards your spouse, or anyone else for that matter, is key. Dr. John Gottman has been studying couples for over two decades at his "love lab" in Seattle. After watching a couple argue or disagree for ten minutes, his group is able to predict with 94% accuracy which couples will divorce or remain married. One of the things they look for is responding to bids for connection. This can be as simple as looking up from your iPad when your wife asks you to look at something. The question we are intuitively asking is, "Are you available when I reach for you?" If you perceive the answer is "Yes," all is well. If you perceive the answer is "No," then that is disappointing. It is the overall pattern of being available that is important, you don't have to be perfect.

Proximity seeking is just that - trying to get close to someone you care about. When we feel attracted to someone, we look for ways to spend time together. (Ever seen those couples joined at the hip?) This is also true when we feel hurt, afraid, or upset. (Not that we as guys will ever admit this). If I have had a hard day or feel frustrated with my kids, then I like to spend time with my wife. She is amazing and I typically feel better just by being around her.

My dog's behavior is a perfect example of proximity seeking. This 60lb black lab mix leaps onto our bed whenever there is a thunderstorm. Something inside of him says that being near me will make him feel safer. Our kids did the same thing when they heard thunderstorms or had bad dreams. After the 9/11 attacks churches were flooded with people gathering to comfort each other and to seek comfort in the Lord.

Guys are more likely to bid for connection and seek proximity through sex. Sex is where we powerfully connect physically and emotionally. If your wife feels like all you ever want is to get lucky, she will not see your advances as bids for connection or proximity.

Knowing about these behaviors helps me understand the Gospel in a whole new way. Repeatedly God is seeking connection with His people through Abraham, Moses, Israel in the desert, the prophets, and ultimately through Jesus. He is the one seeking a relationship with us. He is the one seeking proximity with us, tearing apart the veil in the temple that separated us from intimate connection with Him. Jesus came to seek and to save. He is focused on connecting with us.

Attachment protest is just that - protesting a sense of disconnection. If a bid for connection was missed, or you feel ignored or slighted by someone you love and care about, you will protest. Unfortunately, we tend to be indirect in the way we protest so the message is usually not received. Instead of saying you miss your wife and wish she would spend more time with you, it seems easier to say, "I guess those friends of yours on Facebook are more important than I am." Your wife might say, "You obviously don't care about me or you would call or take out the garbage," etc.

Unclear protests typically feel like an attack or rejection. If my wife says, "You never take out the garbage!" I will dutifully remind her that I did take out the garbage one time back in 2001, and expect a sincere apology for her incorrect statement. A clear protest would sound like this, "I'm really frustrated about taking out the garbage. When you don't listen to me it feels like I'm unimportant to you." Can you hear the attachment significance? It has nothing to do with the garbage, it is all about if I hear and respond to her.

A successful protest is not based on saying the right words or following a certain formula. Teaching couples communication skills is very popular. It sounds like a great idea and there is some value to it if you already have a good relationship. However, studies clearly show that under duress you will not consistently or effectively use these skills. Going to a firing range is one thing. Effectively using a weapon in a combat zone is a different story.

Picking up on the intent to connect is the key. You can totally fumble through what you say or how you say it. If the other person picks up on your intent to connect then things go well. I have watched beautifully-worded attempts to connect in my office but because the wife felt it was an attempt to deflect and was not genuine she withdrew into her shell. I have also seen a guy fumble through an attempt to connect in a painfully awkward manner, but because his wife picked up on his genuine desire for connection it ended up as a beautiful moment.

Sometimes a protest involves withdrawing and getting quiet. Mark came to me after his wife caught him looking at pornography again. Mark avoids conflict like the plague. His wife can get loud and animated when she gets upset or even downright mean. Mark's protest was silent withdrawal. He would avoid being around her (the opposite of proximity seeking) and have minimal interaction with her for a while. His thought processes ran something like this: "I will reconnect with you when things cool down, until then I am maintaining a minimal safe distance." This type of withdrawal is also used as passive-aggressive punishment whereby you are punishing someone with your silence. Both husbands and wives can do this. You are usually well aware when this is being done to you, the silence is deafening. Just so you know: "passive" aggressive is still aggressive.

Repair is when you make up with each other. When conflict creates a sense of disconnection with someone we love and care about, we try to find a way to reconnect. Recognizing and responding to repair attempts will save a lot of heartache and frustration.

Stereotypically, a husband may send flowers to his wife after an argument. Repair attempts are usually much subtler. Making a joke in the middle of a tense discussion, asking how their day was, taking an interest in what they are doing ("What are you watching?" when you can see she is watching HGTV), or doing something nice (getting a cup of coffee, glass of water, etc.). All of these actions can be attempts to repair the sense of connection. This does not mean that the issue has been resolved or that you are admitting that the other person is right. It is simply a sign that you want to bury the hatchet.

Fortunately, repair attempts do not have to be skillfully crafted and executed. It has little to do with what you say or how you say it. Just like a successful protest, successful repair attempts involve the other person perceiving that your intent is to repair. I have watched guys absolutely fumble the execution. They are unable find the right words to say, they say the wrong thing which comes out sounding like an insult. A sitcom writer couldn't create a better script! But as the wife sees his desire to reconnect and willingness to stumble, she softens and they both smile knowing that things will be OK. As you will see later, returning to a safe sense of attachment calms all three brains. Our brains are literally wired for attachment.

My daughter and I were having a tense time due to schoolwork in middle school a few years ago. Things stayed pretty tense and it was difficult for us to talk, but I wanted her to know that I still loved her and cared for her. While she was doing her homework, I would walk over and kiss my daughter on her hormonal pre-pubescent head, and walk away. Once or twice a night I would do this. Things are great now and we laugh about that time. My daughter said she hated it in the moment when I would kiss her on the head, but she also said that it helped her get through that time.

Missing the cue for a repair attempt keeps you stuck in conflict and disconnection longer. When you see repair attempts as off ramps from the freeway it changes everything. These are the moments when the white flag pops out - not for surrender, but for a cease fire. Start watching for repair attempts at home and at work and see what happens.

Let's look at proximity seeking, bid for connection, attachment protest, and repair attempts in action. Lisa is extremely hurt and angry after discovering pornography on Brian's phone again. After a dust-up the night before they are both feeling the tension. The tense silence is noticeable as Lisa reads her book on the couch (probably a self-help book on porn). Brian cautiously approaches Lisa and asks how her day was with the kids (proximity seeking). Her response is short and flat. "Fine, just another day of summer," Lisa says without looking up from the book (rebuffed bid for connection). Brian feels the coolness of her response and decides to push forward. He tells her what the kids were doing outside and makes a sheepish joke about their boys thinking they really are Superman on the trampoline (a repair attempt). Lisa can't hold back a grin since she and Brian have laughed together about this many times. Brian apologizes, "I'm really sorry for hurting you again. It kills me when I hurt you and you pull away. I get why you pull away - it's my own fault" (attachment protest). Lisa softens a bit and assures Brian that she still loves him, and that she is still stinging from last night (successful repair).

They still have work to do. Lisa is still hurting and afraid of letting her guard down again only to discover Brian has returned to pornography. Not all scenarios go this well. I have seen couples massacre each attempt, but as they learn to see what is really going on (the attachment perspective) it changes their whole outlook. There is hope where they could not see it before.

CHAPTER 6:

Attachment And Regulation

Go to www.thepornantidote.com
for additional resources

We are hard wired for connection, for attachment. Your brain literally works best when you are experiencing a safe sense of attachment. When the feeling brain says everything is safe, your thinking brain functions pretty well. It works even better when you feel securely attached or connected to someone you love and care about. Essentially, your brain is "turbo-charged" when you feel connected.

When there is a sense of connection we are at our most creative (a thinking brain function), adventurous (the feeling brain says we are safe), and our bodies are calm and self-repair.

Your immune system is boosted by experiencing safe attachment. The body releases oxytocin, which calms everything down and allows the body to repair itself. In fact, the best predictor of how well someone recovers from heart surgery is whether they are emotionally connected with those around them.

My mom just had quadruple bypass surgery a few months ago. She knew the name of each nurse and technician that came through her room. She knew about their lives and children and yes, they knew all about me when I walked in the room. My mom has a lot of connections in her life, and I think her recovery was shorter as a result of being so connected.

Your brain is designed to regulate emotional and physical intensity. Attachment, the Interpersonal Operating System, provides the ultimate solution for regulating this intensity. Nothing gets all the parts of the brain working together better than a feeling of safe connection. Nothing can hijack the brain more powerfully than an unsafe sense of connection, or perpetual disconnection.

Think about every movie, TV show, book, blog, or commercial that you see. Look for the attachment themes and you will be amazed. It isn't just Disney or chick flicks. In action movies the hero is usually trying to save the life of his wife, girlfriend, or kids. The villain goes after the hero's family knowing the hero will do anything to save them.

In fact, your brain processes attachment as a life and death experience. If you hold a gun to my head, and told me that my wife was leaving me I would feel the exact same thing. A wife that feels betrayed and unloved by her husband, and a husband who is terrified his wife will leave him, makes for a tumultuous and terrifying relationship. Hence the upcoming chapter on married life after porn.

Mirror neurons are a big part of why our brains resonate with attachment. In order to live with and around other people, we need to be able to sense if they are safe or not. A smile and a few platitudes helped the guys in "Oceans 11" and "Eddie Haskell" deceive and manipulate those around them. Mirror neurons help us determine what someone else is up to and what their intentions may be.

Mirror neurons are the part of our brain that observe what someone in front of you is doing. Your brain actually replicates what you pay attention to, in your own body. Don't believe me? Think about this. What do you do when someone you are talking to yawns, or scratches their neck or face? Odds are, if you are really paying attention to them, you will do the same thing.

Still not convinced? Think of any guy that has watched "America's Funniest Videos" and seen the dad take a baseball bat to the groin (NEVER get near a blindfolded 5-year-old intent on crushing the piñata). What does every guy do upon seeing the trauma to this particular male region? He bends over and groans in pain as if it happened to him. That is mirror neurons at work.

Here is how God designed this sophisticated monitoring system to work. You are watching another person talk to you, walk towards you, etc. Your brain replays exactly what that person is doing in your own body by sending small signals to the corresponding muscles. You don't actually do what the other person does, otherwise watching "Cirque du

Soleil" would put us in the hospital. The muscles don't twitch noticeably, even though they are subtly activated.

The part of our brain that monitors these physical sensations picks up on this feedback and sends it to the higher functioning parts of the brain for analysis. The brain is looking for clues about what the other person is up to.

Let's say that the guy across from you in the meeting scowls the whole time. This one is easy to pick up on. Or perhaps the lady at the mall trying to sell you something seemed pleasant and smiled a lot, but something didn't seem right. You are probably picking up on something that you need to pay attention to. It may be nothing- she may remind you of an ex-girlfriend that drove you crazy - or she might be deceptive. Have some fun and pay attention to how you feel (remember - feelings are feedback) when you are talking with others.

So how does this apply to attachment and pornography? First, mirror neurons are heavily involved when viewing pornography. When you watch porn you are intensely focusing on what is happening in front of you. Your mirror neurons are playing out what you are seeing or fantasizing about. Your body responds like it is actually happening because your brain doesn't differentiate between observation and reality. In your mind, you are having sex with the woman on the screen.

This is what Jesus said 2000 years ago: "...anyone who looks at a woman lustfully has already committed adultery with her in his heart." It isn't just looking at pictures; it is committing adultery in your heart. It is a big deal. This does not mean that looking at pornography is justification for divorce, but it does mean that we need to be pretty careful what we let ourselves watch.

Mirror neurons help us out when we are connecting with someone or repairing the relationship. Couples gazing into each others eyes are actually syncing up their nervous systems in a beautiful way. An apology is received and is healing when it seems like the other person has genuine sorrow. Compare this with the apologies we gave in kindergarten when strong armed by the teacher. Check out the Ted talk by Dr. Jim Coan called *Why We Hold Hands*. It is amazing research that makes this point beautifully.

There is great news about attachment and sex. If you have solid sense of attachment and connection with your spouse, then you will have the best sex. You heard me - connected sex is the best sex. This is based on research, not a Sunday school lesson.

The stuff on TV, in the movies or in porn is not realistic. People that have impersonal, exciting sex with lots of partners over time are not satisfied. Unconnected sex primarily releases dopamine (the "gotta have it drug" in the brain). Yes, oxytocin (the natural opiate that makes everything feel good) is released whenever you experience an orgasm. The more connected you are, the more oxytocin you release, the more satisfied you are. However, if you masturbate or have a lot of impersonal sex, then oxytocin levels go down when you orgasm. The feeling of calm and satisfaction doesn't last and you quickly start looking for the next fix. It takes more and more external stimulation, more provocative or extreme porn, to get you aroused. Your wife is not going to want to act like a porn star, and this leaves you feeling unsatisfied.

This is a nasty cycle that makes it easy to retreat into pornography. After all, the women on the screen never say no, they are always happy to please you, and they always affirm you with their looks and their bodies. It becomes too easy to sacrifice real connection with a wife that loves you for the fantasy on the screen. It is the apple in the Garden of Eden all over again.

There is good news. When you and your wife push through to deal with the pain, to rebuild trust, and to both feel connected in the marriage, this is where you find the best sex. This is a way of life that does not drive you to search for a way of escaping reality. Reality becomes something you want to be around for. You want to protect the joy and peace you experience in your marriage. This beats a life focused on "Just don't act out" any day.

I tell the guys in my counseling practice that this is what they can look forward to. Most of the time they look at me as if I just spoke Chinese. Sean was like this. He has been looking at porn for so long that he could not imagine life without pornography being a constant companion.

Then it happened. After addressing things from an attachment perspective and seeing the Lord bring healing to those wounded places, the unthinkable occurred. Sean sat in my office with a perplexed look on his face and said, "It isn't worth it anymore." Sean described how he pulled up porn on his phone a few times over the past week. "It isn't a rush, it isn't exciting like it used to be. Even while I was looking at it, I knew it wouldn't make me feel better in the end. It soured the water for me." He was relieved. He told me how much he was enjoying the freedom from shame and guilt. The weight he felt after acting out wasn't a constant drag.

Sean noticed how he was more available to interact with his wife, his kids, and his friends. He didn't know what he was missing before. Truth be told, Sean didn't think that it was possible to really enjoy connecting with others. Now, Sean is working to stay clean because he likes how it feels to be clean. He is protecting a life characterized by peace and meaningful connections. This is attractive - it pulls him forward instead of trudging along.

The guys I work with repeatedly tell me how much better it is to have hope and work towards something, to protect a life they are enjoying more each day, than simply trying not to mess up. Abstaining from looking at porn or acting out is where you start, but life gets depressing if that is your highest goal. When you are enjoying a sense of life and vitality, the freedom of feeling alive and not looking over your shoulder, looking at porn doesn't make sense.

Before, it seemed like the best option all of the time. Now, it is like asking you to poke yourself in the eye with a stick. That is freedom. That is what the Lord has in store.

CHAPTER 7:

Porn:
Counterfeit Attachment

Go to www.thepornantidote.com
for additional resources

A counterfeit is never as fulfilling as the real thing. However, if we can't get the real thing we start looking for substitutes: Rolex watches for $50 on Times Square, knock-offs of your favorite brands, you get the idea. Sometimes, we are so desperate that we are willing to let ourselves be seduced into believing that something fake is authentic.

When I was in middle school, Panama Jack shirts (yes, I am that old) were all the rage. You had to have one or you were considered lame. We didn't have the money to get a real Panama Jack shirt, so I had a knock-off. Everyone knew it wasn't the real deal, but at least I got credit for trying. It wasn't satisfying to wear it to school, it simply helped keep me from feeling even more rejected. Middle school is brutal.

The news reported that truckloads of counterfeit Panama Jack shirts had been confiscated by the police in New York City. Folks that bought the fake ones walked around knowing that they were wearing a lie, hoping that no one found out.

"Nice shirt!" from your friends was met with a wry smile, knowing that you have duped them. "Hey, your shirt feels thinner than my Panama Jack," provoked a panic that you had been found out, followed by you having to devise some story, yet another lie driving you further into hiding.

Porn is just another example of the enemy offering an apple, a baited exchange of a counterfeit for what is true. What is empty for what is filling. Boy, is it tempting.

God's design for us is connection - healthy attachment. This is the essence of the Gospel. He came to seek connection with us while we were His enemies. We are the Prodigal that He is running to embrace. He is the One pursuing us. That is good news.

Once we took the apple, it created disconnection. We immediately began hiding from the Lord and from each other. When God asked Adam and Eve where they were, He wasn't playing hide and seek. Since He is everywhere at all times it would be a pretty short game. He was seeing if they were willing to be honest with Him, to be seen when they felt shame. We have been doing the same dance with Him and with each other ever since.

Healthy connection provides a safe refuge. Psalm 91 says, "He who dwells in the shelter of the most high will rest in the shadow of the Almighty…" When hard times hit, feeling like someone is with you and that they have your back helps get you through.

Finding out your child died in a car wreck, that your spouse is leaving you, that your parents are divorcing, or that you lost your job – in each of these cases, having someone walk with you through the valley of the shadow of death is vital. Research shows that prisoners of war are much more likely to survive if they feel a sense of connection with another person. For POWs, the survival number is two. Even "The Lone Ranger" had Tonto.

Porn provides immediate escape and numbness. The NFL player getting shot up with Novocain before games is anesthetized against the pain. It does not repair the injury. In the end, it causes more damage.

Surely you have heard about players suffering from the effects of repeated concussions. Escape and numbing lead to more hiding, leading to more isolation and pain, which leads to more escape and numbing. It is a wicked spiral.

Genuine connection is both exciting and satisfying. When she likes you back the two of you can't spend enough time together. You can talk forever and not get tired - it is exhilarating. Likewise, reconnecting with a close friend or relative is both stimulating and comforting. You walk away feeling refreshed and better about yourself.

Porn is the ultimate roller coaster ride. It is super stimulating, and the neurobiological cocktail released in your brain is literally mind blowing. Once you have felt the transcendent high, it entices you to replicate the experience. Your brain can spot a counterfeit - it knows this experience is artificial, and so you are left unsatisfied and wanting in the end. The solution? More porn.

You look for more intense and edgy material to regain the original rush. You look for hours to find the right picture or video to finally masturbate to. Your reward? Shame and exhaustion the next day because you stayed up until 2:00 a.m. on a work night.

Connecting with others you care about, those folks you have a secure sense of attachment to, improves relationships in every area of your life. You become more attuned to others around you. You find yourself knowing what to do in situations that used to cause you stress or lead you into conflict.

I see this happen all the time. Repeatedly guys tell me stories of how their marriages radically improved. They have deeper relationships with their kids, even their co-workers. One of my favorite stories has nothing to do with pornography, but everything to do with connection.

Bob and his daughter Judy were estranged for almost a decade after a bad divorce. Bob regrets all of the ways he hurt his kids and ex-wife in the process. Judy wrote her father off as the devil himself. Over several years Bob reached out to Judy, and she finally agreed to meet with him in my office. It was tense, but what followed over the next year and a half is nothing but miraculous.

Not only have Bob and Judy been able to build a friendship, but the way they see the world around them has radically changed. Judy had become convinced that you cannot trust anyone – after all, if your own dad will burn you then who can you trust? Her best defense was a good offense.

After a lot of work repairing their relationship, they consider each other close friends. Judy can now see that everyone else is not a mortal threat. She can let her guard down a bit and enjoy life, and people, like never before. Bob finds himself seeing people at work differently. If someone is frustrated or stressed, Bob wonders what may be going on in their life instead of discounting them. He is more compassionate and understanding. He likes his new perspective a lot. Risking to connect literally changed the way they see life and (in Judy's case) live life. It is a thing of beauty.

Porn numbs out this sense of connection with others as people and trains your brain to objectify those around you. You tune out relevant emotional and relational information, and experience the consequences. Things get harder, not easier. When I have spent time connecting with my wife or a good friend I end up feeling better about myself. Not because they are building me up, just by being with them. This is how secure attachment works.

Simply being with folks you are attached to impacts you this way. It is affirming. They see me, they know me, they genuinely seem to like me. We are drawn to people like this, and we usually only have a handful of folks like this in our lives. When my wife tells me she loves me, is glad she married me, that I am strong and sexy, I eat it up. Because she really knows me, these sentiments carry some serious weight.

Porn offers the same idea, but wrapped in a fantasy. The women on the screen always want you, they always affirm you, they always long for you with their eyes and their bodies. They are always pleased by everything you do and never say no. The woman on the screen doesn't know you or see you. Her message is everything you want to hear, but it is hollow.

Once you leave the fantasy world on the screen (or in the strip club, massage parlor, lunch with an affair partner) the hollow affirmations evaporate. Reality kicks in. From euphoric high you move to a crushing low. Better make sure that your seatbelt is securely latched and that you keep your hands inside the ride at all times.

Our brains literally resonate with attachment, like a finely tuned Ferrari, Peyton Manning throwing short routes over the middle, or a perfectly tuned orchestra. It is a thing of beauty - all three brains working together in perfect harmony. We are at our most creative, flexible, courageous, and happiest when we experience secure attachment with someone we care about.

Porn throws a monkey wrench in your brain. It makes you numb and paranoid. When you have to hide your phone, delete your history, and make sure all of the files or emails are hidden, you can never really rest. Somewhere inside you know that your sins will find you out. Hoping it will never happen to you provides no rest.

Hiding your phone from your wife is a major tip-off. I can't tell you how often wives tell me that hiding your phone makes them worried and suspicious. It is kind of like having several kids across the house that have been making noise all afternoon who suddenly become quiet. Too quiet. You become suspicious and start investigating what is going on.

So why do we do it? Why do we fall for the same old trap, the same old apple? Especially since you swore to never do it again after how bad it got last time.

Connection is so wired into who we are that we can be easily seduced by the counterfeit. An approximation of the same feeling seems to be better than nothing.

Think of it this way. On one side of a see-saw you have safety. On the other side you have connection. You have to risk one for the other, there is no connection without risk. Risking to connect means risking rejection, abandonment, even humiliation.

If the risk seems too great, we will sacrifice connection for safety. Alone and safe easily sounds like a better idea than risking and feeling worse about yourself. In this case, safety has weighed down the see-saw and left connection hanging in mid air. Safe does not feel alive. "Safe" offers protection from the possibility of emotional and relational death. The absence of threat does not mean you feel alive, not even close.

To be fair, we are called to protect our hearts (Prov. 4:23). It is not a good idea to put your whole heart out there for everyone. There are some people you need to keep at a safe distance. David figured this out with King Saul once the king decided used David for target practice with his spear.

Even when King Saul apologized, David never went back. Wise man.

When we actively resist trying to connect with others over time, we are left with an ache inside. The emotional brain is experiencing the lack of needed connection, which is then conducted to the body brain and experienced physiologically. There is a vast buffet of options to help escape the awareness of this ache: Porn (of course), anger, food, alcohol, workaholic, gaming, obsessive exercise, etc.

Risking to connect can feel like watching trapeze artists at the circus. The person being thrown from one swinging trapeze artist to another can be caught or dropped. The flyers are as calm and confident as can be. They are 100% sure that they will be caught, that the other person is ready, willing, and able to catch them. We can risk when we know we will be caught. Risking to connect, to find someone ready and available on the other side is amazing. This can be a friendship, spouse, a family member.

Just like porn leaves you wanting more porn, connection makes us want more connection. When I eat a chocolate chip cookie (especially a warm one just out of the oven) I want another one. Safe connection inherently makes us feel good and wanting more of this same feeling. Connection and attachment, unlike pornography, comes without all of the negative side effects.

Ironically, when you experience safe connection you feel safe. Remember, the brain harmonizes and resonates with a sense of secure attachment. The emotional brain not only feels safe, it feels some level of euphoria (dopamine and oxytocin).

Connection creates the very safety we need and desire. It creates the safety we need in order to pursue more connection. The more you connect with those you love and care about, the deeper the emotional tie. These are the anchor points that get us through the tough times, and give us courage to reach for more in life. These attachments are your safety net.

Now, the connection side of the see-saw carries more weight. This leads to more connection, which decreases the need for as much safety, which leads to risking for more connection...you get the idea. The sense of safe connection with those closest to you typically spills over into the rest of life: Job, hobbies, and other relationships.

Porn is just the opposite. Porn drives you to hide. You think, "If others see me for who I am and what I have done they won't want anything to do with me." Hiding leads to more hiding. This too spills over into the rest of your life.

You choose which snowball to have rolling. One leads to feeling alive, the other to feeling dead. Refusing to choose is a choice in itself.

Chapter 8:

Connecting With Christ –
The Ultimate Antidote

Go to www.thepornantidote.com
for additional resources

I was so angry at my wife. I can't remember why, but I remember that I was really frustrated and couldn't stand it. Anyone that has ever met my wife wouldn't believe I could be mad at her.

I paced while praying and talking out loud to the Lord, telling Him exactly what I thought and felt. That morning, it was on. I was giving Him an earful, letting God know exactly how mad I was at Julie, exactly what she had done, and how wrong she was. I was on a roll, and it felt good.

The more I poured out my thoughts and feelings to the Lord, the better it felt. I felt like He was encouraging me, saying "Alright, what else do you have Carl....? And then what...? Don't hold back." My pacing became stomping and my arms were waving as I expressed my disdain, and then it happened. God hijacked my prayer.

Just as I was hitting the crescendo, words came out of my mouth that I did not intend to say. My words focused on how He needed to deal with Julie. After the case I just made, surely God had to agree with me. Instead, these words came out of my mouth, "Lord, deal with me first, and deal with me hardest." It felt like I had been shot.

Stunned, I realized the Lord would honor this request. You know that feeling when you say something stupid and you want to grab a fishing pole to reel the words back in? I knew there was no way to undo what I had just prayed. Stunned, shocked, and eerily relieved, I sat there. After ranting for 15 minutes I was silent, humbled, and thankful.

I knew the Lord prompted this prayer and that it was good. He answered the prayer for sure. It humbled me and changed me. It made me a better husband, father, and friend. And it would not have happened if I had not ranted and raved first.

I would not trade this intimate moment with Christ for anything.

Several years before this, I was offended by something Julie said or did as I walked in the door from work. We had two small children at home, so her day was filled with the unending responsibility of taking care of their needs while keeping a constant eye on them. A few hours of that exhausted me. She did it every day.

As I was changing my clothes, I went over what she said in my mind. I became angrier each time I thought about it. In that moment something hit me. I stopped, took a deep breath and prayed, "Lord, what is your perspective on this?" I paused and listened.

A tangible peace came over me along with the thought, "Carl, this has nothing to do with you." With that, I was able to walk into the kitchen with a loving attitude and help my wife.

Both of these scenarios demonstrate the ways in which the Lord wants us to connect with Him. He longs for intimacy with us, that is why Christ came - so that there would not be anything to get in the way of a close, intimate connection with the Lord Himself (Heb. 4:16).

Both of these moments occurred because I poured out my thoughts, attitudes, and feelings to the Lord. I am not giving God new information. God is not turning to Gabriel with a look of shock saying, "Can you believe that!?!" I am pouring my stuff out so that I am ready to hear the Lord.

This is not some kind of formula. I spend time with the Lord in many ways - including reading, meditating on scripture, journaling my thoughts on scripture, etc. However, when I feel strongly about something - if I am upset, angry, afraid, or hurt - it helps me to pour this out in a concrete way to the Lord. Then I am better able to tune in to what He wants me to do without fighting my own thoughts and feelings.

My wife and I taught this at a marriage seminar. A couple came back to tell us how the husband had used it the next Sunday morning. Rick was frustrated and angry with his wife over something that happened that morning. He walked outside and told the Lord exactly what he was mad about and why. Then Rick asked the Lord for His perspective. The anger pretty much evaporated. No major revelation, but he had peace. Rick was a guy that could simmer in his anger, so this was a big deal.

I have told many of my clients the story of "Deal with me first and deal with me hardest." A number of guys have taken the challenge. One man wrestling with sexual addiction recently dared to pray this and told me what a huge difference it made in him, and in his marriage. They are still working hard, and their marriage is better because he dared to pray in this way.

Praying this way is not about letting the other person off the hook. It is about taking the log out of your own eye before confronting someone else. When I have needed to confront my wife, or anyone else, talking to the Lord about my anger first has always been a good idea. When I act out of my anger, no matter how "just" it may seem, it always blows up in my face. When I deal with the Lord first, my prideful anger and bitterness don't rear their ugly heads.

Another incident that highlights this way of dealing with the Lord in the moment occurred several years ago. I was flipping through the channels one night looking for a football game when I ended up seeing something sexually explicit. I think it was a free month of HBO. I wasn't looking for it. I didn't want to see it, but it was already in my brain.

The image was intense and my flesh wanted to camp out there. I can not tell you how often the guys I work with tell me about these kinds of situations - seeing a commercial, someone pushing an iPhone in their face with porn on it...it isn't fair.

Frustrated that I had been ambushed, a thought hit me. I can't unsee what just happened, so I asked the Lord to remove the intensity from what I had just seen. I sat there for a moment and something amazing happened - it worked. Because the intensity was gone, there was no struggle with lust or intrusive recall of the picture. This is gold. This is freedom. As I have shared this with my clients the results have been amazing. There is an escape route when you see something - you do not have to be in bondage to it. The relief these guys talk about is awesome to see and hear.

Taking it one step further, I have challenged men to think about the worst times they have acted out - looking at porn and masturbating at home or work, going to massage parlors, prostitutes...you name it. As they recall these events there is a lot of shame, fear, and lust. The challenge is to picture Jesus in the scene with you, and ask Him to help you connect with His presence.

The shame shoots to surface immediately. "It is so awful, I can't think of Jesus there," they say. Ever since the Garden of Eden, shame has driven us into hiding. This can be gut-wrenching as these men prepare for the condemnation and judgment they anticipate is coming their way.

Just the opposite happens - they experience peace and forgiveness. Now Jesus is the most compelling feature in that scene of their life. There is nothing to hide from, and nothing to feel ashamed of. Nothing intense to lust after. I challenge you to try this with something in your life. Recall the event, feel the emotions connected to the event, and picture Jesus there. When I do this, I ask Jesus to help me experience His presence. He is everywhere at all times, even if I did not pick up on it the when the event originally happened. This has been a very healing experience for me, and for the folks I work with. Try it and see what happens.

Everything I have described in this chapter is a way of intimately connecting with Christ. If attachment is the antidote for sexual addiction, then attachment with Christ is the ultimate antidote. He is always available. He is always loving. He is always compassionate when we turn to Him.

All that I have described in the past chapters about emotions, the three brains, and attachment applies to our relationship with Christ. He is the One who is seeking us out. Intimate connection is the reason Jesus came as God in the flesh in the first place. Too often I feel like God is disappointed in me, upset with me, or too busy to focus on me (what with the starving kids in Africa, earthquake and tsunami victims, etc). Instead, I believe that the best illustration of how the God that created the universe loves us is – wait for it - Pepe Le Pew.

If you don't recognize the cartoon character of Pepe Le Pew then check it out on YouTube. Trust me, it is worth it. As a skunk, Pepe is always chasing down the cat with a white stripe down her back. Pepe, with his thick slick French accent, perpetually chases after her.

Pepe never gets angry, never throws up his hands and gives up, he never stops - ever. Pepe is always spewing his affections as he chases after the cat, who is constantly running, hiding, or pushing him away. For the few moments Pepe gets to hold the cat he kisses her and gushes about her beauty and how he wants to whisk her away. She runs, and he is only more in love with her.

What a beautiful picture of being passionately pursued by Christ. No matter who you are, or what you have done, this is how the Lord is pursuing you. It is time to let Him catch you and hold you.

CHAPTER 9:

Caught Red-handed – Her World Falls Apart

Go to www.thepornantidote.com
for additional resources

"**Y**ou have to see me NOW!"

This is the call I receive all the time. "My wife found porn on my phone (iPad, laptop, etc). Then she found out how long I have been looking at it. You have to help me save my marriage!" She has been asking on and off to go to counseling over the past few years, but now he can't get an appointment fast enough.

Crisis has a way of focusing us and motivating us. Ironically, I pray for the perfect crisis when things are really stuck. If you are in a crisis like this, rest assured - the Lord is not fretting or sweating. He often allows a crisis in order to break things loose.

If you are reading this and you are married and struggling with pornography, then you probably know what it feels like to be found out. Rarely do I get a call from a guy saying that he felt guilty and decided to tell his wife that he has been viewing pornography. It goes so much better when you confess rather than wait until you are found out.

When a wife discovers her husband has been looking at pornography, a bomb goes off inside of her. Sometimes it is nuclear. The greater the shock to her, the greater the impact. If your wife has no idea that porn has ever been a problem for you, she will be pretty devastated. Here is the shocker: What you have been looking at is not the biggest issue. Read that sentence again. The images and videos are not the greatest threat to her. Betrayed trust is far more wounding than looking at porn and masturbating, or even meeting women in real life.

Wives wonder who they are married to. "Who is my husband, really? The guy who leads Bible studies, is a Deacon, volunteers with the youth, and may even be a pastor himself, or the guy who seeks out porn, lusting and feeding his mind with this stuff?" This conundrum literally fries her brain. The whole experience is traumatic for her. No one is shooting at her, planes did not crash into a building in front of her, but it is trauma nonetheless.

Trauma is an overwhelming emotional experience that leaves us feeling inherently out of control - helpless. Life seems to come undone. Therefore it affects every area of our lives. Essentially, if you thought life was going along fine, and then something overwhelming happens, you readily start questioning how stable everything else is. She is perpetually waiting for the proverbial "next shoe" to drop.

Combat veterans with PTSD describe trauma very well. The helplessness of watching buddies die, or being trapped and sure they will die are described as traumatic. The same is true with kids who find out that their parents are divorcing. They may have known that there were problems, but now their whole world is rocked. Their naive trust that things will work out gets ripped away, and their whole view of relationships is dramatically changed.

This experience is quite different for her and for him. Let's start with what the guy is going through- there is trauma for him as well.

FOR HIM

Whether you are caught for the first time, or caught again, something is going to hit the fan. It is messy and it does not smell good. You are experiencing a swirl of shame, terror, anger, and confusion. Partial confessions are a dime a dozen at that moment.

Your wife is already angry, crying, and yelling over what she already knows, so telling her more will only make it worse, right? But trying to convince your wife it is an isolated incident, something that just began recently, or that she is making too big of a deal out of it are panic behaviors, akin to trying to put out a campfire with gasoline.

Be sure to read the next section to learn what not to do when disclosing your history of looking at pornography or other sexual betrayals. Seriously, this is crucial. There is one mistake that can set you back months, especially when you repeat it. So read carefully.

Typically, there are two ways guys react here. First, they might become aggressively defensive. Guys try to convince their wives that they did not really find anything. If this applies to you, you will try to talk her out of her reality, even telling her that she is crazy or a prude. Either way, you further betray her trust and dig a bigger hole to save your own hiney.

Tactic number two is terrified damage control. Your wife's intense emotions are overwhelming and so you assure her it will never happen again, that she caught it at the very beginning, and you will do anything to fix the situation. Promises of marriage counseling, getting more involved at church and men's groups, and using internet filters flow.

"As long as no one else finds out we will get through this," you may think. The seed is planted for the next episode. Just as Adam and Eve immediately hid in the Garden, so the pattern of hiding is perpetuated. Only bad things grow in the dark.

After numbing out with porn for so long, the pain and fear are overwhelming, with no readily available escape. Afraid of losing his wife, his reputation, his image, perhaps his job, a guy in this situation feels incredibly helpless. Remember, helplessness by itself is an amazingly powerful trigger for acting out behaviors.

Unfortunately, these promises don't typically last. Once the crisis lessens so does the strength of his commitments. Attending the men's group becomes less of a priority. He gets irritated when she checks his phone ("It feels like you are treating me like a child," he says). Attending church as a family starts to slide again.

Three weeks and three months are typical breaking points. Without the fuel of a crisis or active support from others who know the truth and love you, it is a matter of time before things break down again. Each time the cycle repeats everyone becomes increasingly numb and more detached. It is no longer a matter of dying in a house fire. Instead, the result may be slow death by asphyxiation.

The best thing you can do in this situation is to get connected with a group of men that know the truth, love you, and will walk with you. Going it alone is a death sentence. Again, even The *Lone* Ranger had Tonto.

FOR HER

Your wife has a very different experience. While you have been hiding porn, you have known about it all along, and that you could be discovered. Often, the guy experiences great relief because he is not hiding all of the time but now the secret is out. This is not the case for her.

First, recall that porn does not make sense to her. Women who look at pornography usually do so to make a guy happy, and so they go along with it. They don't like it and they do not "get it" because their brains are wired differently.

She will not understand why you fail to think about your wife and children while looking at pornography. She does not have the same experience in her brain when seeing something sexually provocative. In fact, she can not fathom how you could not be thinking of the impact on your family in that moment.

To be fair, consider the female equivalent of pornography, cutting and eating disorders. Most guys do not understand these behaviors. Sure, some guys struggle with these behaviors, just like some women struggle with pornography, but the majority of guys would not dream of starving themselves when feeling overwhelmed or out of control. Obsessing about calories and fat content just does not make sense to most guys - just eat and get over it, right? For women in that struggle it is an all-out battle.

If this is the first time she has discovered pornography, it is devastating. Each time she finds it again she feels like it is an affair - not just voyeurism, but an actual affair. Pornography is the other woman. Or in this case, thousands of other women that she can not compete with. They are airbrushed. They are a fantasy that no one can compete with.

Fantasies never have a bad day, whereas your wife will. A fantasy always wants to jump your bones, whereas your wife will not. A fantasy is only focused on making you feel good, no matter how tired or stressed she is. A fantasy never has to refrain from sex because of her period. Your fantasy is the other woman, and it is time to break things off.

If she has discovered porn repeatedly (every few months, every year or two, every few weeks) it becomes a raw spot.

"How many times do we have to go through this?" she screams. Your wife is afraid that this will keep happening for the rest of your marriage, which is supposed to be the rest of her life. Imagine living with a guillotine over your head that can drop at any time. It gets old fast.

Chances are she may have known something was up because you have been coming to bed later, or pushing the boundaries in bed, or not as interested in sex. Typically your wife knows something is wrong. Knowing the truth provides some relief, because she no longer has to wonder.

The trauma created by betrayed trust can be consuming. I call this a "hair on fire" experience. In the moment, the pain and fear are overwhelming. She feels like it will never end. The feeling brain is in the driver's seat and it is in full on panic mode.

Your wife is likely to make some dramatic statements like, "I can't keep doing this," "I can't stay married to someone that does this," and "What kind of pervert are you?" These cut deep, and it is hard not to take them personally. Her hair is on fire and she is flailing about trying to make it stop. It can be brutal.

Recall that our brains process attachment in the same way as life and death experiences. When our most important attachments are threatened the whole world comes apart. That is exactly what she is experiencing when the person she loves and trusts the most is the same one that has ripped her heart open and deeply betrayed her. You are simultaneously the source of pain and comfort for her. This is an irresolvable conflict that has smoke coming out of her ears.

The helplessness from the shock of discovering porn, that she could not see it coming, prevent it from happening, or prevent it from happening again, is traumatic. Remember, the deception is worse than the sexual sin. That wound goes deeper. How do you love and get close to someone that you do not trust? Or worse, when you are not sure who they "really" are?

Josh Duggar, star of the reality show following his large family in the upper Midwest, was found to have molested one of his sisters. He also had several affairs, betraying his wife. He was on the Ashley Madison list published on the internet. Now his own sisters have said that they do not know who he really is. How can the same guy they see at Thanksgiving be the same guy that does this stuff? It can be horrifying to say the least.

When this process repeats itself, a predictably miserable cycle begins with her discovering porn (or chatting with women, your name on Ashley Madison, another email account linking you to a dating site, etc.). You feel incredibly ashamed and sincerely make every promise in the book with an oath on your mother's grave to stop forever. Somewhere inside you know you won't keep it.

Things calm down and the two of you start getting along and having sex again. Your motivation wanes and life kicks back in. The sting from the last meltdown is gone and the fuse is burning down until the next explosion. Couples that I meet with report years of living like this. The cycle may take a few weeks, months, or even years to repeat. Every time it does something dies inside of her.

Your wife starts protecting her heart from what she feels will inevitably happen. Not knowing drives her to put up protective walls around herself. If she does not feel safe giving you her heart, she will not feel good about giving you her body. If you want great sex, you have to protect her heart.

Sex can be quite a roller coaster after the secret is out. Predictably, your wife may want nothing to do with sex for a while. Since porn is the other woman, she does not want to share, compete, or least of all be compared with the other women. In other cases, a wife will become very sexual and adventurous. Be careful - this is a panicked attempt to keep you by being better than porn. This is typically a mad flurry which is very confusing for both of you. Beware - once the panic fades she will probably feel cheap and angry that she has to "perform to win you back."

She may ride the roller coaster of being angry and attacking you, followed by jumping your bones because she loves you and is afraid of losing you. When the cold shoulder comes back around your head is spinning. If this happens you must remember that she is not crazy. Rather, she is traumatized by intimate betrayal. Your wife feels crazy and out of control. Your words cannot comfort or reassure her.

Again, our brains process attachment like life and death. The person you are married to is typically your closest attachment. The rupture of that attachment is called an attachment injury. Imagine a ligament connecting you with your wife. An attachment injury is more than a muscle strain. It is a partial tear in the ligament. If you have ever had this kind of injury you know how painful it is. You know that it does not heal quickly. You know that even when rehab is completed, if you turn your knee just the wrong way and exacerbate the injury, it feels like the injury happened all over again.

This is what your wife experiences when you act out again. Similarly, her pain and trauma are often triggered when she hears of someone struggling with porn, seeing a movie or TV show featuring pornographic content, or anything else porn related.

To make things more complicated, your wife's serotonin levels will also drop. As a result, she will obsess about what has happened and how vulnerable she feels. She will be vulnerable to bouts of anxiety and depression. These can manifest by shutting down or getting angry. Put on your big boy pants, you owe it to your wife to ride the roller coaster that you put her on.

Unfortunately, the trauma and lower serotonin levels means that your wife is prone to invasive recall during sex. During sex she is thinking about sex. I know what you're thinking - "Thank you, Captain Obvious." This means that her brain is making associations with other memories regarding sex. The hard drive pops up with what she thinks you were looking at, and her sex drive comes to a screeching halt. If this happens, know that this is not voluntary. It is invasive recall, which is common with trauma.

Anniversaries can be dicey the first year after things come out. If the problem is ongoing then it is a lot harder. Your wedding anniversary, the anniversary of when she first found porn on your phone (or when your kids found it on your phone and told mom) – these are all hard for her.

The same is true for places that are now associated with sexual betrayal - restaurants, cities, stores, parks, etc. You can be having a great day together when a commercial for one of these places derails the whole evening.

To be fair, in this situation there are typically other marital problems in addition to problems with pornography. Problems in the marriage can fuel the emotions that make you look for an escape. If your wife is constantly critical and demeaning, this will need to be addressed after things have stabilized and there has been some healing. Until then, she will have a hard time hearing about anything she has done that has hurt you. Especially if there is any implication that she has pushed you to act out or look at pornography.

Make no mistake - you are 100% responsible for looking at porn. However, you are both responsible for creating an environment that makes either one of you want to escape from each other.

A lot of the work I do is with couples who want to repair the damage after sexual betrayal. Too often, the guy wants to tell his wife it is her fault for making him turn to porn because of what she said or did that hurt or made him angry. I reassure him that we will get there, but that it isn't the first concern we will address.

Ironically, most wives are relieved in the end to know that there is something they can do to influence the situation. At first it is hard, because she feels like all of the blame is being placed on her. Once she sees that something she is doing hurts her husband, it provides a whole new interpretation of his behavior. Seeing him hurt or feeling fear invites a loving and sensitive response when she feels safe.

This is a game changer.

CHAPTER 10:

Spilling The Beans –
All Of Them

Go to www.thepornantidote.com
for additional resources

Would you rather endure a brief but brutal beating, or death by a thousand cuts over several months? Most of us would rather get the beating over with rather than endure torture over a prolonged period of time. Your wife would agree.

Whether your wife caught you or you decided to come clean, your best option is to spill the beans. Spill all of the beans. You are not protecting her by giving her the highlights and skipping over the details. She is going to be mad, she is going to obsess, and she is going to ask lots of questions to try to make sense of everything. More details will come out.

As I have already said, we tend to give out information a bit at a time. "I am trying to spare her from dealing with so much at once," you may argue. This may be your motive to some extent, but another part of you hopes she will not ask any more questions. You hope you will not have to reveal all of what you have done, so you keep hiding.

Trickling out the truth over time is like re-opening a gaping wound with the revelation of each new detail. The wound never has a chance to heal. Your wife gets stuck in anger and numbness. She is always waiting for the next shoe to drop.

You are not doing your wife or yourself any favors by trickling out these details. If you want to prolong the healing and recovery process while eroding any level of trust you may have built up, then the trickle effect is a great way to do it.

At this point the husbands in my office say, "If she is threatening to leave over what she already knows, then I can't tell her any more…she'll leave me for sure." I really do feel for you if this is the spot you are in. It is truly terrifying.

Recall that deception is more devastating for her than sexual betrayal. Volunteering information actually starts to restore trust. As weird as it sounds, your willingness to be honest with your wife even though it is painful for her and stressful for you, actually rebuilds trust.

Because you are volunteering information instead of your wife discovering it, she can begin to think about letting her guard down. If the primary way she discovers information is from her efforts digging and investigating, she is left with this realization: "I can only trust what I discover...and and there is always more when I dig."

She can not let her guard down and begin to heal if she is always playing detective. Your wife is miserable in that role and needs your help to bring her detective duties to an end. When your wife finds out about your porn use, visits to massage parlors, chatting, affairs, etc., she is in shock. Shock buffers the impact of discovery. This is the most loving and gracious time to be totally honest with her.

If you are truly concerned about her well-being then consider meeting with a trained therapist for help and guidance. Do not drag things out. Find someone and go meet with them. Just the fact that you are wanting and willing to be open and honest with your wife goes a long way.

Let's be clear about something - this is going to hurt your wife. It is going to be pretty painful, and yet it is the right thing to do. Hurt and harm are not the same thing. Hurt is when something is painful, yet this pain leads to healing. Cleaning out a cut, getting a shot, soreness after exercising, and even disciplining your kids. All of these involve inflicting pain of some sort that is in the best interest of the person experiencing the pain.

Taking away my teen's iPhone as a consequence of bad behavior is very effective. They may think it is harmful, but it isn't. Harm means the pain is destructive, and that no good will come of what you are doing. Beating your children, telling them they are no good, and targeting a quarterback's knees - all of these are destructive and have no redeeming value.

Hurt will seem like harm because your wife may react strongly with shock and anger. Once she knows the truth she can begin processing and grieving it. This is where you learn to ride the bronco. Some guys have been riding the bronco with a wife who has bipolar disorder, or something else that keeps her upset or depressed a lot of the time. This will need to be addressed and dealt with as well. That will come later.

Focus on the crisis at hand, and take responsibility for your behavior and your choices. Your wife may be verbally abusive. This may explain why you turn to porn, yet it in no way excuses it. Man up and own it. Be aware that she will be on this roller coaster for a while. Commonly, guys get impatient and upset when things are not stabilized or feeling normal within a weak or two. Typically the guy wants it all to go away because it is too stressful and he feels guilty. He starts trying to shame or bully his wife into being quiet or "getting over it."

Yes, you told her. Yes, that helps. No, it does not completely restore trust or give you the right to shut her down. Admitting to robbing a bank does not mean that logical consequences are removed. You owe it to your wife to walk through this with her. Just don't do it alone.

Now for the million dollar questions: What to tell your wife? How much to tell your wife?

For starters, give her the 1,000-foot view. Tell her what you have been doing (looking, meeting folks, etc.), how often, and where these things have occurred. If there are people involved that she knows, or places that affect her, she has the right to know. I cannot tell you how often affairs happen with a close friend of a spouse. Bottom line - she deserves to know, so rip the bandage off quickly.

Some wives want a lot of details: What did you look at, what types of things did you get into, where did you meet women, what did you do with them, what did you say in your chat sessions. Some wives do not want those details in their heads. She may go back and forth between these two stances.

She gets to decide how much detail is revealed. This is tricky, since once your wife knows something she can not un-know it. The more details she knows, the more questions she will have. Sometimes she will get stuck, always wanting to know more details which then sends her into a spiral of fear, hurt, and anger. If this happens you should seek help from a professional marriage counselor with experience in this area.

Here are some guidelines that may help if you are getting stuck in this situation. Once there have been a few weeks following full disclosure and the questions keep coming, see if she will agree on a 24-hour delay. If she wants to know more details she can ask. Both of you pray about it for 24 hours. After 24 hours if she still wants to know, then you should tell her.

Understand that your willingness to share these details, to be honest, is just as important as the information itself. If your wife understands that you are willing to be open with her, verses withholding information to protect yourself, then she will have some relief. Trust is being restored.

Beware of a deadly pitfall as you disclose information to your wife. If you step on this landmine you are guaranteed to scoop burning coals into your own lap. The landmine that wreaks havoc: Protecting the emotions or identities of those you acted out with. Decide if you want to remain married. If so, your wife's feelings are the only ones you really care about.

If you had an affair you will have compassion for the woman you were with. You will not want to harm her. You will be tempted to defend her as a good person. However, you can not serve two masters. As Jesus said, you will love one and hate the other. The fantasy of the other person has to die.

Your wife has the right to try to contact people, which can set off a fire storm. So be it. They chose to play. You can choose the behavior, but not the consequences. Again, if you are concerned about your wife's response, seek professional help for the marriage. You can not trust your own judgment regarding what is right in these situations. As for your wife, I can assure you that she will not trust your judgment.

I highly recommend seeking the help of a Christian counselor with training in this area. Specifically, I recommend seeking out someone trained in Emotionally Focused Therapy (EFT). EFT is the most empirically validated form of marital therapy by a long shot. EFT provides an effective roadmap to navigate this marital minefield in a way that leads to healing, rather than mere survival.

Both of you are going to need support. Do not foolishly try to do this on your own. We are so prone to clinging to the image of having it all together. Avoiding the shame and embarrassment of being exposed is just as destructive as hiding porn.

You are burdened with keeping up the image while you are dying inside. How many times have you heard of a couple that seemed like they "had it all together" announce they are divorcing?

I have always found it amazing the way we put on a great front at church. We may be arguing and fussing on the way to church. Once the car doors open the Holy Spirit hits us and we are doing great - until we get back in the car. We have all done it.

Finding a group is essential. I like Celebrate Recovery, an all-purpose support and recovery group with chapters throughout the country. It provides structure for safety, and allows folks to be the body of Christ for each other. There is no charge to attend. Celebrate Recovery has been a huge blessing for the husbands and wives I work with.

Coming out of hiding is essential for both of you. Hiding makes the problems worse. Try going to a group like this for a few weeks as an experiment. The guys I work with say it has been a huge help. They support each other and feel loved no matter how they have behaved.

God has amazed me as I work with men and marriages affected by pornography and sexual betrayal. He has shown me how He never wastes pain. Pain makes us aware of our need for Him. As we turn to Him, He provides peace and guidance as we learn comfort from being totally dependent on Christ. Romans 8:28 says that He will work all things together for good for those who love Him. It does not mean that what happened was good, but that the Lord who created and maintains the universe is actively working in your situation to bring something good out of it.

Isaiah 61 says that He will exchange "Beauty for ashes, joy for mourning, and praise for despair." This is what I watch the Lord do. This is what keeps me coming back to work each week.

Couples that choose to turn towards each other and towards Christ end up with better marriages than if nothing ever happened. This is the brass ring, and it is available for you. I beg you to go for it.

CHAPTER **11**:

Recovery For Him, Her, And The Marriage

Go to www.thepornantidote.com
for additional resources

Recovery is learning to do life differently. When you have been living a life focused on pornography, or managing life by escaping into porn and sexual addiction, changing how you deal with life is a big task. As you have heard me say repeatedly, this is one task that you should not try on your own.

Doing life differently means coming out of hiding. Coming out of hiding about porn and sex-related behaviors is where you start. Lasting change requires you to go deeper into the wounds, fears, and beliefs that keep you in bondage to your iPhone.

Refusing to look at these emotional drivers means that your "recovery" will be short-lived. It will either go dormant as the guilt and shame subside, or you will simply jump to another addictive behavior. It happens all the time. Guys trying to stay away from porn find old vices popping up with a vengeance: Alcohol, gaming, eating, smoking, etc. Those that try to go it alone are the ones that struggle the most and typically give in. Once again, even the Lone Ranger did not go it alone.

Coming out of hiding means telling other people what you have been doing, and telling them in detail. This is not a discussion for Sunday School. Find a group of guys who struggle with this, or other similar issues, and put it all out there. One guy I work with prefers going to A.A. instead of a sexual recovery group.

"Do I have to tell others?" is a question every guy asks. The same answer applies to everyone, and that answer is "Yes." The secret keeps you in bondage. The fantasy of protecting your image becomes more important than getting better or protecting your wife and family. Jesus said that if something causes you to sin, cut it off and get rid of it (Matt. 5:29). If it is your eye, then gouge it out. If it is your hand, cut it off. If it is your smart phone, get rid of it! In other words, do whatever it takes so that it is not easy or convenient to continue destroying yourself and others.

James 5:16 bluntly states, "Confess your sins to each other." Why? There is great power in coming out of hiding. Every guy I work with is afraid, most are terrified, of telling others. You would think someone has a gun to their head. Once they take the risk and tell someone they experience amazing relief. Literally they come back telling me it feels like a physical burden has been lifted from their backs.

It will not feel right at first. You will look for a million reasons not to tell anyone. The enemy does not want you to come out of hiding, because hiding keeps you isolated where he can steal, kill, destroy, and torment you with fear, shame and guilt. Take a deep breath, then just do it. You are only as sick as your secrets.

Coming out of hiding means doing life with others. Really doing life with others. Fantasy football, tailgating, and neighborhood cookouts do not cut it. You need people in your life that know your story, and you know theirs. Where you are honest and real with each other when things are going well, and when everything seems like it is falling apart. Jesus had a closer relationship with Peter, James, and John. He didn't go it alone, so why do you think it will work for you?

There are a lot of different support groups out there. Some even meet online, which opens up a world of options. If you are struggling primarily with pornography, and the vast majority of your acting out has been alone and in secret, then I recommend Celebrate Recovery.

Celebrate Recovery is an all-purpose support and recovery group created by Rick Warren. Men and women meet separately and there is always a small group for men addressing addictive behaviors, including sex and porn. This is usually the largest small group.

Typically, the guys I work with who have experienced the greatest changes have been involved in Celebrate

Recovery. You can find a group near you at www.Celebrate Recovery.com.

Sexaholics Anonymous (S.A.) and Sexual Addicts Anonymous (S.A.A.) are versions of A.A. that specifically address sexual addiction. In my experience, guys that attend these groups are further down the line of sexual addiction. They are much more compulsive and have had much more contact in person to hook up for sex. Guys that struggle primarily with pornography consistently tell me that the leave these meetings more triggered than helped.

There are a lot of other groups that are catching on across the country, and some only exist in certain areas. Look into these groups and try one for a few times. Yes, showing up to a group for guys openly acknowledging that they struggle with pornography and masturbation is awkward. So is your wife or child walking in on you masturbating at the computer, or finding the videos and images left behind.

Everyone talks about accountability. There is a need for accountability, in the context of support. If accountability is simply behavior checking it will not last because it is legalism. The law always brings death (Rom. 7:10).

This is where the groups are powerful because everyone is in the same boat. Some guys are much further down the path of recovery. Some guys have traveled much further down the path of addiction. There is no shaming or guilt-tripping there since everyone knows what it is like to fall, and what they need when they fall. It is simply amazing to watch this in action.

Groups like this are where you find safe people to reach out to when you are tempted or triggered. Talking to someone that will give you a lecture, sermon, or a blank look is not what you need. You need someone who knows what it is like to be really tempted in this area. They will know how to pray for you, how to support you, and how to lovingly confront you.

"What about internet filters and accountability software?" you may ask. I am asked this question all the time. Before going into specific options, you need to be clear about the purpose of these tools. They will not keep you from looking at pornography, they will simply make it more difficult. No filter can catch 100% of the threats unless you only want access to Sesame Street and Barney.

Filters are speed bumps to slow you down. They keep you from impulsively setting off a neurobiological bomb in your brain that can flash into a raging forest fire in a heartbeat. There is always a way to beat the system. For most wives this knowledge may not be reassuring, but it is necessary to know.

Filters are a great idea for everyone. They keep us and our kids from intentionally or accidentally coming across material we do not need in our minds. That means having filters and/or accountability software on all devices with internet access including cell phones, tablets, laptops, PCs, iPods, etc.

Work computers are often the weak link. Understandably, employers want to keep unnecessary or harmful programs off of their computers. Some companies have their own filter. Even then, there is always a way to beat the system. I have worked with a number of guys who have lost good paying jobs, including prestigious careers as officers in the military, because they were looking at pornography on the job. That is proof of the power of porn.

If you are really struggling with the temptation to seek out and view pornography, and your cell phone is the weakest link, then switching to a "dumb phone" may be your best option. Yes, it is humbling to whip out your flip phone from circa 2003. It is more humbling to lose everything that you value to keep up the appearance of having life under control. If your iPhone causes you to sin, cut it off.

Recovery involves changing your marriage as well. Learning to do life differently means that you and your wife are learning to do marriage differently. After all, when two become one, whatever you do affects your spouse.

This means coming out of hiding as a couple. Both of you need other people that know what is going on. No more hiding, no more secrets. Wives wring their hands over not wanting embarrass their husbands by telling anyone. They also avoid their own embarrassment, and cling to the façade, telling themselves that "Everything is OK."

She needs someone to talk to, to vent to, to cry with. She does not need to tell the world or post everything on Facebook. She does need some girlfriends to walk with her through the blood and the mud. If she does not it will all come out on you, and it will not be pretty. Yes, you may have a hard time looking her friends in the eye, but this is a necessary sacrifice.

Marital recovery means riding the roller coaster while you each adapt to, and create, a new normal. Unfortunately, both spouses often feel like they are doing this with their hair on fire. It can be pretty rough.

Devastating pain and paralyzing fears that you will lose your marriage and family, or things will never get better, seep into every area of life. I highly recommend finding a marriage counselor experienced in helping couples through this type of crisis. As I mentioned previously, I have been trained in Emotionally Focused Therapy and I believe this is an incredibly effective model for helping couples recover.

Coming out of hiding in your marriage means your wife gets unrestricted access to your cell phone, texts, email (all email accounts), Facebook, Twitter, Instagram, etc. In some cases your job may entail dealing with classified information that would keep you from sharing emails with your wife. If that is the case, then I recommend finding someone at work for accountability.

This is where I commonly hear a lot of pushback. "I'm not a 12-year-old, I don't need mommy checking up on me. It's humiliating!" That is your pride speaking, and you need to swallow it whole. Since you have betrayed your wife's trust you have the responsibility of earning it back. Being there and providing for the family helps build trust, but it not sufficient. You have to build back trust in the areas where you betrayed it.

Did you delete your history? She needs to see your history. Did you chat or exchange emails with a woman? She needs to see your emails. She does not trust you for a good reason - you have not been trustworthy. Fighting transparency only makes you look and sound like you are still acting out. Maybe you are. Resisting being transparent, or guilt-tripping your wife by accusing her of not forgiving you and never wanting to trust you is shooting yourself in the foot.

Imagine that you own a company and your best friend since elementary school is the chief financial officer. If you caught him stealing tens of thousands or hundreds of thousands of dollars over the years, how would you feel? If he said, "I'm glad you caught me. The guilt was killing me. I promise I'll never do it again," would you believe him? Would you fire him? If you kept him on, would you check the books to make sure he doesn't do it again? You know you would. So don't whine about natural logical consequences. They stink but they are necessary.

If you have been meeting women or stopping by strip clubs, then your wife may want to be able to track you on your phone. She wants to trust you and she is terrified of being made to feel a fool again. If she wants to track you, which will be humbling, the best response is a loving "Yes dear, if that will help you." The more she looks and sees that you are where you said you would be, the more she can let her guard down. Push back indignantly and all she thinks is, "He is still acting out and he doesn't really care about me." Pride kills. Let her track you and prove yourself to be trustworthy.

Your wife's recovery will be different than yours. Guys typically experience relief when the truth comes out, but her hair is on fire. She may be relieved to finally know what has been going on. However, dealing with the emotional reality of your deception, and what you have been looking at, can be a shotgun blast to the chest for her.

Unfortunately, this can re-ignite occurrences of betrayal in her past: Parental divorce, molestation, rape, infidelity, etc. Instead of just dealing with the current situation with you, she is emotionally dealing with wounds from her past as well. Like re-aggravating an old sports injury, it isn't simply a choice, but a natural response.

One in three women have been touched sexually in a way they did not want by the time they reach eighteen years of age. Lots of kids have had their world come apart when their parents divorce. Chances are your wife has some wounds that you just stirred up.

Telling her the truth is still the right thing to do. Lying to her for her own good is lying to her for your own good. Fortunately, God is very efficient when it comes to pain and crisis. He exposes everyone involved exactly where He wants to deal with them in order bring healing. Not management, but healing.

As things stabilize and the emotions are not as overwhelming, as your relationship becomes safer and you can really hear each other, she will recognize her faults in the relationship as well. It seems we all have logs in our eyes. Her faults will never justify your behavior. However, they do provide some insight. Ironically, the wives I work with tell me that seeing their part gives them more of a sense of control - there is something they can do.

Take care that your wife doesn't interpret this to mean that it's all her fault. It's dangerous if she starts thinking things like, "It's all my fault because I...", or "The pressure is all on me to..." These are deadly lies that are too often planted by the husband.

If your wife yells at you and degrades you in front of your friends and family, while refusing to have sex with you for four years, you cannot blame her for your behavior. She helped create a problem and has to take her fair share of the responsibility. However, your behavior is your choice and yours alone. Own it and life will go better for you.

Cutting, eating disorders, and shopping are the female equivalents to pornography. Women and girls are much more likely to resort to these behaviors when feeling overwhelmed or out of control. These behaviors create similar changes in the brain as those caused by looking at pornography. Most guys do not understand these any more than women understand porn.

Remember, the function of any type of addictive behavior is to manage or escape stress. Typically, the stress comes from a sense of shame, hopelessness, or helplessness. Dealing with the root causes while connecting intimately with Christ and others is the ultimate antidote. Do not get stuck on playing "Behavior Police." It will drive everyone crazy.

Getting stuck in anger is a common pitfall for wives when there is betrayal. Fear of getting caught off guard again and being devastated makes anger an attractive bunker in which to hide. Just telling her to let go of her anger will blow up in your face. Acknowledging her fears, and acknowledging that you have given her good reason to be afraid, means your wife will be more likely to step back from her anger.

Sometimes the power of always having the upper hand is too much to pass up. You will know this is happening when anytime there is a disagreement or conflict, your wife will reach for the "But you looked at porn" trump card. The same thing happened with Adam blaming Eve in the Garden. It did not work then and it will not work now. It is a sticky issue to confront, and it needs to be addressed.

Relapse and collapse are different. Relapse is repeating old behaviors while you are struggling to deal with the root causes and connect with others. Relapse is a part of recovery. Read the last sentence again. Every week guys come into my office frustrated, mad at themselves, and feeling hopeless after acting out again. Each time this is an opportunity to dig in and see what was really triggered and deal with the root causes. The relapse is not something to celebrate, but exposing your own sense of being wounded and going on to find healing is.

Guys will be doing well, and then they seem to impulsively revert to looking. This reveals what has or has not changed in them. I love it when they look at me with a sour look on their face and say, "It just wasn't worth it, it isn't like it used to be." That is reason to celebrate. The old stuff is losing its attraction.

A collapse is completely reverting to the old pattern of behavior, or even going deeper. This is giving yourself over to lust and reveling in it. Ongoing binging verses a slip and fall. This is very much a dog returning to its own vomit.

Relapse is painful, but a collapse feels devastating. Either way, Christ takes us by the hand and keeps walking with us. Because of Him there is always hope - hope for you, your wife, and your family.

Being connected with others is vital. Christ and others become your anchor points. If you fall, they help you keep from falling too far. They help dust you off and lift you up again. Both you and your wife need this. In fact, you were made for it.

RESOURCES:

Internet Filters and Accountability Software:

Covenant Eyes www.covenanteyes.com

XXXwatch www.XXXchurch.com

Open DNS www.opendns.com

*filters at the router level

Groups:

Celebrate Recovery: a Christ centered support and recovery group for hurts, habits, and hang ups with groups throughout the country. www.celebraterecovery.com

Sexaholics Anonymous: www.sa.org

Sexual Addictions Anonymous: www.saa-recovery.org

Check for independent groups in your area.

Intensives:

Bethesda Workshops: intensives for men, wives, and couples.

I have personally observed one of these weekends- it is worth your time and money.

www.Bethesdaworkshops.org

Mark Laaser's workshop for men:

www.faithfulandtrue.com

Recommended Reading:

Healing the Wounds of Sexual Addiction Dr. Mark Laaser

The Betrayal Bond: Breaking Free of Exploitive Relationships Dr. Patrick Carnes

Safe Haven Marriage Dr. Sharon Hart Morris May

ABOUT THE AUTHOR

Carl Stewart earned his MA in counseling at Denver Seminary. He is a counselor and coach in an overflowing practice working with men and marriages devastated by pornography and sexual addiction. He has advanced training and supervision in Emotionally Focused Therapy- the most empirically validated marital therapy which is uniquely suited to restoring marriages affected by sexual betrayal. Carl Stewart is a paid speaker at men's events, marriage retreats, and parenting seminars.

To learn more about Carl Stewart, go to:

www.thepornantidote.com

www.carlstewartLPC.org

Made in the USA
Middletown, DE
13 July 2018